AF691727

# AI *Curbside*

*The Practical Guide for Busy Clinicians*

Kirk D. Wyatt MD, MAS

# Frontmatter

Copyright © 2026 Kirk D. Wyatt. All rights reserved. No part of this book may be reproduced, stored in a retrieval system, or transmitted in any form or by any means—electronic, mechanical, photocopying, recording, or otherwise—without the prior written permission of the publisher, except for brief quotations in critical reviews and certain other noncommercial uses permitted by copyright law.

Library of Congress Control Number: 2026910640

ISBN 979-8-9958402-0-6 (hardcover)

ISBN 979-8-9958402-1-3 (paperback)

ISBN 979-8-9958402-4-4 (ebook)

ISBN 979-8-9958402-3-7 (audiobook)

Published by The Curbside, LLC, West Fargo, North Dakota

thecurbside.ai · aicurbsidebook.com

For permissions, errata, and inquiries, contact kirk@aicurbsidebook.com

First edition

## Disclaimers

The views expressed are those of the author and do not necessarily reflect those of his employer or research collaborators.

Nothing in this book should be construed as medical advice. This book is intended for educational and informational purposes only and describes the author's personal experiences and perspectives on the use of AI tools in healthcare workflows. Clinical decisions should always be based on a licensed clinician's own professional judgment, institutional guidelines, and the specific circumstances of each patient. The author and publisher disclaim any liability arising from the use or misuse of the contents of this book.

Nothing in this book should be construed as legal advice. AI is an emerging field abounding with uncertainty. Be sure to comply with all applicable laws, policies, and procedures as you utilize AI tools. As I will highlight in this book, AI can be a powerful tool, but you—the user—are ultimately responsible for how it is used and applied in the world we live in.

Many of the AI products described in this book are proprietary, and their inner workings are not always fully transparent—even to advanced users. Tools that appear similar on the surface may behave quite differently under the hood, and individual products evolve frequently. Descriptions in this book reflect my personal understanding of how each tool worked at the time of writing, based on publicly available information and my own use. Nothing in this book is a guarantee or warranty of how any specific tool currently functions. Always consult the vendor's current documentation, their terms of service and privacy policy, and your own institution's policies before using these tools.

The AI landscape is rapidly evolving. Parts of this book are likely to be out-of-date by the time you read it. While I've done my best to ensure everything in this book is accurate as of the time of this writing, I'm sure some lingering errors remain. If you identify any of these errors, please accept my apology and then email me at kirk@aicurbsidebook.com so that I can address them in a future edition.

## AI Assistance

Portions of this book were drafted, edited, and refined with the assistance of a variety of large language models. Cover artwork was developed with AI assistance. The author reviewed all content, made all editorial decisions, and takes full responsibility and accountability for the final text.

## Financial Disclosures

Potential financial conflicts of interest related to the content in this book include the fact that I receive royalties for copies sold on all platforms (including ElevenReader and Amazon, which I mention in the book). I have received research funding from the Chan Zuckerberg Initiative through a sub-award. EvolutionaryScale, which is discussed in Chapter 18, was acquired by the Chan Zuckerberg Initiative. I have participated in usability testing and provided feedback to the UpToDate team on their Expert AI feature. No financial or in-kind compensation was exchanged for participation.

## Trademarks

Product names, logos, brands, and other trademarks referenced within this book are the property of their respective trademark holders. Use of these names does not imply endorsement.

# Table of Contents

# Prologue: I Used AI to Write This (and I'm Still Accountable)

Let's get the elephant in the room out of the way.

I used artificial intelligence to help me write the book you are reading right now. I'm telling you this up front, not as a gimmick, but in full transparency. I didn't use AI because I'm lazy. I used it because I am a full-time pediatric oncologist and clinical informatician with a wife and two young children. Like you, my time is my most fiercely guarded resource.

AI didn't do the work *for* me. I didn't just tell it "write a book on AI for physicians" and use that for the book. I worked *collaboratively* with AI through a lengthy back-and-forth process over seven weeks to develop the ideas, write the text, go through several iterations of revisions, copyedit the text, and develop the logo on the cover. AI amplified my work. It helped me put out better work, faster.

Here's a concrete example: as I listened to a draft of the audiobook narrated by an AI voice as I did chores around the house, I would quickly jot down rough notes on things I wanted to change—a phrase that sounded awkward, a point that needed clarification, a factual claim I wanted to double-check. I then fed those rough (and messy) notes to an AI model along with the full manuscript and asked it to find each quote, describe the problem, and suggest a revision. I reviewed each suggestion, accepting some, rejecting others, and revising many. The AI did the tedious work of locating passages and proposing fixes so that I could review and edit the book on the fly, and I made the editorial decisions. That workflow—human judgment steering AI capability to improve the quality and efficiency of work—is precisely what this book teaches.

Another motivator for using AI is that if I had written this book the traditional way—from start to finish, completely from scratch during spare time on evenings and weekends—it would have taken me months to get a draft to a publisher. In the AI space, 12 to 18 months is a lifetime, so by the time you got around to reading it, much of what is in this book would be outdated. It would be a historical artifact.

But here is the most important thing you need to know: *I* am ultimately accountable for every single word, idea, and recommendation in this book. I used AI as a tool to help me write better and as an accelerator to help me write faster, but the ideas are genuinely mine. If there are mistakes in here (as I'm sure there are), they are my mistakes, not the algorithm's. In the end, you can be the judge of the final product—is this book just a bunch of "AI slop," or is it a polished book that helps you meaningfully improve your life? Did AI degrade the quality of the book, or improve it?

In this book, I'm going to break down how these tools work in terms you can understand. I will show you how I use AI in my day-to-day life as a physician and researcher, and explain how you can practically apply AI as a busy healthcare professional. My promise to you is simple. By the time we finish our brief time together, you won't just understand the hype around AI. You will get hands-on experience with a practical, actionable framework for how to use it safely and effectively in your daily life—starting today.

# Part I: Getting Started

# Chapter 1: AI Is Here

## Your Use Is Optional. Your Exposure Isn't.

Medicine is, by design, a conservative profession. We are taught to be skeptical of the "new and shiny" because, historically, the "new and shiny" hasn't always been proven to be safe and comes with many unknowns. We demand evidence, we demand trials, and those things take time.

This is, in part, why healthcare has lagged in adopting and leveraging exciting new technological advancements. Major technology companies have become impressively adept at using data spread across public databases and left behind as crumbs of our internet browsing history. They're so good at this that they can show us targeted ads that we'll reliably click on (and make them money in the process). If tech companies are so good at this, why can't healthcare be so savvy? Why can't we put these algorithms to good use to improve human health, instead of reducing the role of this technology to tempting us to buy things online that we don't need?

With the emergence of **generative AI** (that is, artificial intelligence that generates novel content) over the past few years, things are changing rapidly. AI is now one of the most powerful general-purpose technologies that have ever existed, and it can be wielded by anyone with plain-language prompts. It's now everywhere: AI is here, whether you like it or not.

My hope is that if you are reading this book, you're curious about AI and looking to seriously use it in your everyday life. If you're one of those people, congratulations! You are ahead of many of your peers.

If you're still skeptical and hoping AI will just go away as a passing fad, I hope that I can convince you in these pages that you risk being left behind. I'm not saying I think AI is going to replace you in your job; instead, you will be outpaced by your peers who are using it and—crucially—using it *better* than you. I want you to protect your time, your relevance, and your agency. I want *you* to be the one who stays relevant because you've effectively wielded these tools. That's what this book is about. I'm going to teach you everything you need to know to integrate AI into your workflows to help you put out better work, faster, and hopefully reclaim some personal time in the process.

## Reps Beat Theory

If you take one thing away from this book, follow this advice: the only way to understand what AI is truly capable of is to use it. Use it early, often, and on a variety of tasks.

You cannot learn to be a doctor just by reading a medical textbook. That's why medical training doesn't end in the classroom —it takes years of clinical rotations, residency, and for many, fellowship to develop the judgment and expertise required to care for patients.

You cannot learn to use a **large language model (LLM)** by just reading articles about it. You have to get behind the wheel. When you use it daily for low-stakes tasks, you start to develop an intuitive sense for its strengths and its limitations. This will help you feel more comfortable using it for more advanced and complex tasks. If you make these tools part of your everyday workflows, through that process you'll understand the good, the bad, and the ugly.

As you build confidence, you'll discover that the real power isn't in asking quick questions—it's in having AI do complex and time-consuming tasks for you. AI can generate custom briefings, help you analyze datasets, build slide presentations, and even write code to create tools you didn't know you could build. It's those things that will be the real game-changers in how you use AI.

## Don't Drive Last Year's Model

Before we go any further, we need to discuss a small investment I'm going to ask you to make. There are free versions of AI tools, and there are paid versions. If you're one of the growing majority of Americans who have used an LLM, you're probably saying, "I already have enough subscriptions I don't use. Why would I pay for this if I can get it for free, and it already does what I need?"

If you are using the free version of these services, you need to understand that you are driving last year's model. Actually, in AI-years, you might be driving a car from a decade ago. Or, if the vendor lets free subscribers access the current model, it provides only a small amount of usage—just enough for a test drive.

The companies that built these models reserve their smartest and most capable models for their paying subscribers. The models provided in the free versions are relatively inexpensive to operate, but they hallucinate more often, and they don't reason as well. If you're using these models, you are not experiencing what today's AI can do.

You might be hesitant to spend your hard-earned money on an AI subscription. After all, you're probably still trying to pay off your student loans. But as a busy clinician, if an advanced model saves you just thirty minutes of administrative grunt work a week, the money you invested in that subscription will be repaid many times over. You don't realize what you're missing out on until you use the most advanced **frontier models**. Consider the paid subscription a professional investment.

In a short while, we'll be rolling our sleeves up and testing out some different models. This AI speed-dating exercise is going to cost $5 (I'm keeping the stakes low for the skeptics). After that, you'll have tried several models developed by different companies and can decide which one (or ones) to subscribe to. More on that in a bit.

## The Mindset Shift

As we walk through the coming chapters, I want you to keep one rule in mind: focus on your workflow, not the tool.

The tools will change. New companies will emerge. The model that mesmerized you last year will quickly become "last year's news" and a new model, developed by a different company, will become the new crown jewel. But the workflow—the process of identifying a bottleneck in your day, passing that task along with relevant context and constraints to an AI model in the form of a carefully structured prompt, and verifying the output—will remain the same. It doesn't matter which model you are using.

There is one more mindset shift I want to plant early because it becomes increasingly important the more you use these tools: *stay mindful* as you use these tools.

When you send a prompt to an AI model, the response streams back to you in real time, word by word at a pace that feels breathlessly fast. I've found that this speed creates a subtle psychological pressure—a feeling that I need to keep up with the machine, fire off my next question before I've even finished reading the last answer, and keep the momentum going. And when you have a paid subscription with a usage allowance that resets every week, you find yourself racing to use as much of that allowance as possible by the end of the week so that none of it is "wasted."

Resist these urges. You are not in a conversation with a colleague who will get impatient if you pause to think, and the model will still be there tomorrow if you don't use it today. The model is obedient. It will wait for you. It has no feelings to hurt and no schedule to keep. Take the time to carefully read what it produced, evaluate whether it's accurate and useful, and *then* decide what to ask next, and don't feel like you have to use AI for *everything*. In our technology-driven lives, we are constantly bombarded with emails, text alerts, and notification popups that fragment our attention and pull us toward mindless reactivity. One of the major criticisms of social media is that while technology initially promised to connect us, some argue that it has degraded our focus and shifted our focus toward performing shallow, distracted, and mindless interactions.

You can fall into this same trap with AI tools if you let them. You ask the model to perform a task, and while it works in the background, you try to multitask—checking your inbox, glancing at your phone, and starting another chat. But multitasking is largely an illusion; what we're really doing is rapidly bouncing between tasks, doing each one worse than if we'd given it our full attention.

As I've used AI more over the past year, I've made a deliberate effort to treat my interactions with these tools as opportunities for *focused* work, not *fragmented* work. When I'm working with an AI model, I try to be fully present in that task—reading its output carefully, thinking critically about what it said, and crafting my next prompt with intention. This is where the real value lies. The clinicians who get the most out of AI won't be the ones who use it the fastest and outsource everything to AI; they'll be the ones who use it the most thoughtfully and collaboratively.

## Key Takeaways

- AI is now a general-purpose technology that every clinician will encounter, whether they choose to use it or not. Early adopters will have an advantage over their peers.
- The only way to understand what AI can do is to use it—early, often, and on a variety of tasks.
- Invest in a paid subscription to access the most capable frontier models; free tiers use older, less capable models that do not represent the state of the art.
- Focus on the *workflow*, not the tool. The tools will change, but the process of identifying a bottleneck, crafting a prompt, and verifying the output will remain the same.
- Stay mindful when using AI. Resist the urge to multitask. Read outputs carefully, think critically, and craft your next prompt with intention.

# Chapter 2: Garbage In, Garbage Out—Prompting as Clinical Communication

Let me take a poll of the specialists in the room (generalists, please don't take offense). You are alerted to a new consult on the hospitalist service. The reason listed for the consultation: anemia.

Anyone who has ever worked on a consulting service understands the frustration of the terrible consult request. You have no idea what the primary team wants based on this one-word reason for consultation. Are they asking you if the patient has anemia? Is this a question about an urgent critical value, or a curbside question about a routine CBC? Did they diagnose the patient with anemia but want to know why? Do they know why, but need help figuring out what to do with it? Are they asking you to take over primary management?

Because the input was lazy and vague, your output—the consultation—may not end up being what the primary team actually needed. A consult should always indicate the reason the consult is being sought—what is the *specific* clinical question? How, exactly, can the specialist help you?

Talking to AI is the same. The more specific your question, the more specific its response will be.

There is a misconception that artificial intelligence is akin to magic—that you can type a half-baked thought into a text box, and the computer will somehow read your mind and produce a masterpiece. I've been surprised by how well AI usually fills in the gaps when I leave them out of my prompts. But if you want

AI to perform at its best for you, understand that if—in general—you put garbage in, you will get garbage out. If you put a thoughtful, detailed prompt into it, you're much more likely to get what you're looking for.

Can you blame it? Let's say I give it a generic prompt, like *"Write a book on how to use AI."* The model needs context to be able to tailor it. Is this for children in grade school? Professionals? What industry do they work in? Are they engineers or creative writers? What kinds of AI use are you interested in? How long should the book be?

Poor performance of AI models when given limited context about the task is not an inherent fault in the model itself; it is a fault in the prompt. The skill of writing instructions for generative AI systems is called **prompt engineering.** It sounds highly technical, but it's really just a fancy way of saying that you've thought carefully about what you want, and you've clearly articulated the ask to the system so that it gives you what you want. There are many frameworks for how to construct a prompt optimally, but I've found they can be distilled into five key components:

1. **Role:** "Who" is the AI pretending to be?
2. **Task:** What exactly do you want it to do?
3. **Context:** What is the background information it needs to know?
4. **Constraints:** What are the rules it must not break?
5. **Format:** What should the final output look like?

**The rule is simple: the more context you provide and the more specific your instructions are, the more likely you are to get what you want out of the model.** While anyone can pay for a subscription, prompt engineering is an *art*, and it's what is going to separate the AI super-user from the AI novice. Careful prompting takes time and thought—this is what I mean when I say that AI can work *collaboratively* with you, but you need to engage with AI with intention. You are the boss, carefully overseeing the operation. You dictate how the work is done, and the worker does it how you've asked for it to be done.

## Tell It What *Not* to Do

When writing prompts, most people focus entirely on what they want the model to produce. But it's just as important to tell the model what you *don't* want. Think of it as setting boundaries. Without explicit negative constraints, the model will fill gaps with its best guess—and its best guess might include exactly what you were hoping to avoid.

Negative constraints are powerful because they preemptively close off one of the model's most common failure modes—making a wrong assumption. Here are a few examples of what this looks like in practice:

- *"Do not rewrite the text for me. Only identify the problems and explain why they are problems."*
- *"Do not use any medical terminology that a non-medical person would not understand."*
- *"Do not suggest changes to the research study that would require collecting additional data."*

## Ask It to Think Step by Step

Another crucial prompting technique is deceptively simple: *ask the model for a structured approach with intermediate checks.*

When you give a model a complex task in a single prompt, it attempts to produce the final answer all at once. This is like giving it a patient presentation and then asking it what the next steps for management are. You'll get a management plan, but you'll lack visibility of the differential diagnosis and the rationale for this plan unless you ask the AI to “show its work.”

Try asking the model to break a complex task into smaller subtasks, state its assumptions, and walk through each one with verification steps before moving on. For example, rather than prompting, *"Analyze this dataset and give me the results,"* try:

> I need you to analyze this dataset. Before you start, break the analysis into logical steps and list them. Then, work through each step one at a time. Show me your work at each stage before moving on to the next.

What's powerful about this approach is that it gives you visibility into the model's “reasoning.” You can review the output of each subtask, catch errors early, and course-correct before those errors propagate into the final result. Maybe the model misunderstands your dataset structure—if you catch it early on, you can fix it before it produces a beautifully formatted but fundamentally flawed analysis in the last step.

This is one of the most effective human-in-the-loop strategies you can adopt. You're not blindly accepting a finished product; you're supervising the work in progress, just like reviewing a trainee's reasoning on rounds—you want to see the thought process, not just the conclusion. The model does the heavy lifting, but you maintain oversight at every stage. Rather than simply handing off work to the model, you are actively *collaborating.*

## A Bad Prompt vs. a Good Prompt

Let's look at the difference between a bad prompt and a good prompt.

Let's suppose you instruct an AI model:

> Improve my grant application.

If you type that, the model will likely give a generic response indicating things that you have done well, things that you could add, and may well strip out your personal voice, leading to a boring and plain application.

Now, let's use our framework for a good prompt:

> Act as a rigorous, highly critical peer reviewer and research scientist (Role). Critique the attached specific aims page for my upcoming grant (Task). The grant is proposing a new tool for identifying sepsis in pediatric patients, and is being submitted for review by the health informatics study section (Context). Do not rewrite the text for me. Point out logical flaws, confusing jargon, and areas where the methodology seems weak. Do not suggest changes that would require collecting additional preliminary data (Constraints). Provide your feedback as a bulleted list categorized by 'Significance,' 'Innovation,' and 'Approach,' and score it on a scale of 1 to 9 (Format).

When you hit enter on that second prompt, you are going to get highly structured, critical, and immensely insightful feedback. Both responses come from the same model and result from analysis of the same grant application, but the second prompt provided specific enough instructions to tell the model *exactly* what you want out of it. Notice how the prompt includes both positive directions in the task (point out logical flaws) and negative constraints (do not rewrite the text, do not propose changes requiring new data). That combination is what keeps the model on track. Crafting these prompts takes extra thought and attention, but as you'll see, the payoff of spending a little extra time on your prompts can be immense.

If you get a response from an AI system that isn't quite what you wanted, your first instinct might be to blame the model, give up, and declare your AI use a failure. Before you do, look at your prompt. Did you give it a clear role? Did you set constraints? Did you tell it what *not* to do? Rather than seeing a disappointing output as a failure and a reason to abandon using AI for the task, see it as an opportunity to clarify the prompt and to iterate on your ask. This is the *art* of using AI that will set apart the average user and the super-user. If you're able to walk the AI model through the steps it needs to go through to coax it to get you what you want, you will be much more satisfied with the output.

I cannot overstate how powerful good prompting is. Later in the book, I'll show you how the major AI platforms now let you save your best prompts as reusable "skills" that you can invoke over and over again. We'll also review how these platforms can keep a memory of previous conversations and ground every response in the knowledge it gleaned from those conversations. When you look under the hood, you'll discover that these sophisticated-sounding features are nothing more than carefully crafted prompts—the same kind of prompts you're learning to write right now. The five-component framework we just discussed isn't just a tip for getting better responses; it's the foundation for building your own personalized AI tools. Master the prompt, and you've mastered the machine.

## Key Takeaways

- Garbage in, garbage out: the quality of AI output is directly proportional to the quality of your input.
- Structure your prompts using five components: Role, Task, Context, Constraints, and Format.
- Tell the model what *not* to do. Negative constraints close off common failure modes and keep the model on track.
- Ask the model for a structured step-by-step approach with intermediate checks—this gives you visibility into its "reasoning" and lets you catch errors early.

# Chapter 3: Data Privacy and Business Sensitivity

## Think Before You Copy and Paste

Now that you know how to talk to AI, we need to pump the brakes for a second.

In healthcare, we are uniquely burdened by privacy regulations. In the United States, the **Health Insurance Portability and Accountability Act of 1996 (HIPAA)** strictly limits how and when patient data can be shared. And while you probably know better than to paste a patient's name and date of birth into a random website, the risks with generative AI can be a bit more insidious.

Let's start with a basic assumption: if you are using a free version of a large language model, you should assume that your inputs may be retained and used for model improvement unless you've verified otherwise. As a colleague of mine likes to say, "If the product is free to you, then *you* are the product. Your data is the payment for use." The defaults vary by vendor, region, tier, and account settings, but in many consumer-grade AI tools, the use of your data to train models is opt-out, not opt-in. Before relying on any tool for sensitive work, check both the settings and the privacy policy to confirm that training is off, and that data retention is limited. Before you enter any data into a tool, you *must* understand how the vendor uses your data.

HIPAA includes a very specific list of identifiers. If you remove those identifiers and have no *actual knowledge* that remaining information could be used to identify the individual, your dataset may subsequently be considered de-identified under

HIPAA via the Safe Harbor method. The problem is that this does not mean that the patient cannot be re-identified at all.

Let's consider a hypothetical example. You practice pediatric oncology in Fargo, North Dakota. Frequently, families will post about their children's journey on social media, and sometimes patients' stories are picked up by the news media. Let's suppose a 2-year-old with a very rare type of cancer is seen in the clinic. If you were to enter into a large language model the patient's age, the cancer type (a rare presentation)—and the model understood the context that you practice in Fargo, North Dakota—even if identifiers are removed, rare combinations of details can be re-identifying. If prompts are stored or reviewed by the vendor, linkage to publicly available information becomes possible, potentially compromising the patient's privacy.

A contrarian may say, "Well, you removed all the identifiers, and it was the family's decision to post on social media. If they were so worried about re-identification, they shouldn't have shared on social media." The issue here is that the family carefully selected what information they wanted to share publicly. If you share additional information with a generative AI model that the family wished to keep private, this information may be incorporated into the model, violating the patient's right to privacy.

So, what is the solution? How do we work with LLMs in productive ways without compromising patient privacy?

First, you should know, understand, and comply with your employer's policies regarding use of generative AI and all applicable laws. While many employers have strict and stringent policies about how you can use AI—and these policies may feel constraining at times—know that these policies are there to protect you, the institution, and your patients.

Some organizations enter into a **Business Associate Agreement (BAA)** with one or more AI vendors. This is a legal contract between the organization and a vendor that requires the vendor to protect patient data in accordance with HIPAA. Enterprise contracts that include a BAA typically include terms prohibiting the vendor from using your organization's data to train its public models. With the appropriate agreements and terms in place, an organization can legally and securely share information with the vendor under HIPAA.

The ideal situation is that your hospital provides an approved AI tool under a BAA. However, even in cases where a BAA is in place, you should take care to only include the minimum necessary amount of **Protected Health Information (PHI)**.

If you are considering putting identifiable information into an LLM, be sure to check with your institution about the contract. Just because the vendor *can* enter into a BAA doesn't mean that one is in place with your institution.

Now that we've talked about PHI, we also need to talk about sensitive business and academic information.

Let's say you have an incredible idea for a research grant. You've spent months drafting the concept and feel confident that it will get a fundable score. To leave nothing to chance and ensure your proposal is well-polished, you drop your final draft into a consumer-grade, data-training-enabled LLM to check your grammar and spelling. At the very moment that you upload that document, you are handing your intellectual property to a tech company.

Now, your arch-rival research lab on the other coast asks the LLM to come up with a new research idea. The LLM returns a brilliant concept that is, in reality, a carbon-copy version of your idea that it learned by training on your data. They are awarded the grant, and you just got "scooped."

If you are using a consumer account, I recommend that you dive into the settings and explicitly **opt-out of the vendor using your data to train models**. This is usually euphemistically referred to as something positive like "help improve the model" but really, what it amounts to is "use my private data for free to improve your product." Most paid tiers (and some free tiers) allow you to opt-out, ensuring your chats are never used to teach the next version of the model and ensuring the data you put into the model doesn't become the output another user sees.

The rule of thumb is simple: if you aren't comfortable sharing it freely on the internet, do not paste it into a consumer AI tool without ensuring that you have turned off data training and you fully understand how the vendor uses your data. For processing of PHI and business-confidential information, ensure you are following your employer's policies and all applicable laws and only entering PHI in cases where the transfer of PHI is covered under a BAA.

Privacy isn't a reason to avoid AI. It is just the guardrail that keeps us on the road. Now that we know how to steer, and we know where the rails are, let's peek under the hood and learn how this engine actually works.

## Key Takeaways

- Never enter protected health information (PHI) into a consumer-grade AI product. Ensure that a Business Associate Agreement (BAA) and appropriate security protections are in place, and always follow your organization's policies and procedures before entering PHI or business-confidential information into an AI tool.
- Assume your inputs may be retained and used for model improvement, unless you have verified otherwise in both the settings and the privacy policy.
- Even de-identified data can be re-identifying when rare combinations of details are combined with publicly available information.
- Opt-out of data training in your AI tool's settings.
- Privacy is not a reason to avoid AI; it is the guardrail that keeps you on the road.

# Part II: How AI Works

# Chapter 4: The Clinician's Mental Model of LLMs

You don't need to be a physicist to order an MRI. You don't need to know the complex mathematics of radio-frequency pulses or spin echoes. But you *do* need to know enough about how the machine works to understand why a patient with a certain type of metal implant cannot go inside it.

The same rule applies to AI. You don't need to be a software engineer or a mathematician to use LLMs. But you need to understand the basic mechanics of how they process information or else you will trust the model when you shouldn't, and you will get frustrated when it fails in totally predictable ways.

In this chapter, we'll build a simple, practical mental model of what an LLM actually is, and more importantly, what it is not.

## It Is Not a Database of Truth

When we use Google or UpToDate, we are searching through a digital filing cabinet. We type in a search term, and the system retrieves links to specific, pre-written documents that (hopefully) contain the answer to our question.

An LLM does not work like this. At its core, a large language model is simply a sophisticated version of the autocomplete feature on your smartphone. It has ingested mountains of text—articles, books, websites, and research papers—and built a complex statistical map of how human language fits together. When you ask it a question, it is not "looking up" the answer from a definitive source of truth. It is calculating the statistical probability of the next word, over and over again, at lightning speed.

Let me give you a couple of examples. I'm going to start a sentence, and you fill in the blank:

*The cat has very pointy ...*

What did you say? Maybe you said ears, or teeth, or perhaps even claws.

Let's try that again:

*The cat has a very pointy ...*

What did you say this time? Tail? Nose?

The LLM can pay *attention* to the fact that the word "a" significantly changes the meaning here—it suggests that the body part "pointy" is describing something that the cat only has one of. For that reason, the statistical probabilities of various words coming next are different, all because of this one-letter word. This *attention* mechanism is the foundational innovation of the Transformer architecture that today's LLMs are built on.

The LLM doesn't *know* the answer. And really, there isn't a single "right" answer to many questions you might ask it. But the LLM knows what a correct answer *looks like*—in this case, it's going to be referring to *some* body part that cats have that comes to a point. This is an incredibly important distinction that we will come back to when we discuss why these models sometimes invent things out of thin air.

## Correlation, Not Causation

A subtle but important point: AI models learn *correlations*, not causal relationships. When an imaging model flags a chest X-ray as showing pneumonia, it hasn't learned how to make a clinical diagnosis. What it has learned is which arrangement of pixels is statistically correlated with images that radiologists previously labeled "pneumonia" in its training data.

Take a more pointed example: imagine a model trained on chest imaging where chest tubes happened to appear disproportionately in patients with cancer—not because chest tubes cause cancer, but because malignant pleural effusions are a common reason to need a chest tube. The model can latch onto the chest tube itself as a shortcut for the cancer label. Now imagine that model encounters a new patient who has a chest tube placed for a complicated pneumonia. The presence of the chest tube nudges the model toward "cancer," even though the chest tube has nothing causal to do with the diagnosis. The model isn't reasoning about cause and effect; it's correlating. That distinction is critical.

But this same property is also one of AI's greatest strengths. AI's real superpower isn't replicating a single, obvious pattern that a clinician could find in a textbook—we're already pretty good at that. It's pulling signal out of problems where there is *no* single dominant feature, just many faint, interacting signals that, taken together, drive the prediction. This is where AI quietly outperforms humans, and it's a useful mental model both for spotting good AI use cases and for evaluating whether a tool you've been pitched is solving a problem AI is well-suited for.

## Embedding

I'll try not to get too technical, but I'd like to explain how language patterns and the meanings of similar words are encoded in these models.

Have you ever used a music recommendation service like Pandora, where you give it a song you like, and it creates a "station" that plays similar songs? How do these systems work? Early versions of Pandora utilized a "fingerprint" for each song that was manually coded by trained music analysts for the Music Genome Project. The idea here was that there were a variety of specific musical characteristics that could be graded in their strength in any song. Let me give you a few examples of the types of things that you might see in such a model:

- Country music
- Rock instrumentation
- Strong female vocals
- Christian religious theme
- Syncopated rhythm

Consider hundreds of attributes like this that could be rated on a scale of one to ten and rated for every song.

Now, think about how you might plot the strength of a given characteristic on a graph. Let's start with a one-dimensional line graph of "Country music" that puts very traditional country music closer to ten. On this line, songs close to a ten have a strong "Country music" sound, and ones at zero sound nothing like "Country music." Let's now add a second dimension: "Rock instrumentation." Now we have a two-dimensional graph, where each song can be represented as X and Y coordinates for these attributes—say with country music on the X-axis and rock instrumentation on the Y-axis. You could see how different styles of country music with rock undertones could be characterized. Let's add another dimension for "Strong female vocals"—now we're working in three-dimensional space. We can place each song on a three-dimensional graph, with its position encoded by a set of X, Y, and Z coordinates. The set of coordinates that pins a song to a specific location in space is called a **vector**.

You can imagine how songs that have similarities in these characteristics will cluster together so that songs that are similar will be physically "near" each other in three-dimensional space. This is precisely what music recommendation tools like this are doing. They will start by playing songs that are very close in "space" to the seed song. As you rate certain songs with a thumbs up or a thumbs down, the characteristics of those rated songs will become more heavily (or less) weighted and shift the center of the space (and perhaps even the size of the sphere of space) from which future songs are chosen. Occasionally, the model may present a song that is a little different to see if you like it. It will use your response to that "stretch" sample to see if it should expand options in that direction or stay clear of that path.

Are you with me so far? Let's consider another example I'm going to borrow from Nikhil Birajdar at towardsdatascience.com. I'll give you a two-dimensional graph with the X-axis representing "maleness" and the Y-axis representing "royaltyness." I have plotted out "King" and "Princess" on the graph. Can you tell me where "Queen" and "Prince" belong?

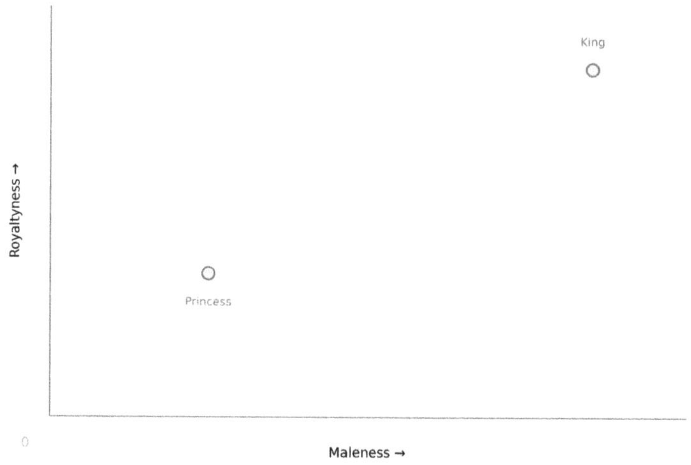


You probably ended up with something like this:

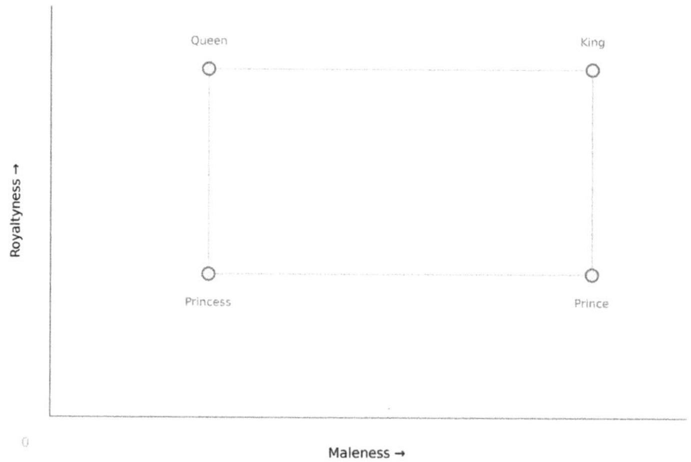


The parallelogram pattern captures word relationships. King→Queen parallels Prince→Princess

Through this exercise, you can see how meaning can be encoded in vectors and that these vectors can become mathematically computable. That is—the numerical difference in the position on the scale of "maleness" between a king and queen is about the same as between a prince and a princess. It may be difficult to conceive, but now imagine that we weren't just limited to three-dimensional space and every word was encoded in a vector of thousands of dimensions. This is how LLMs encode meaning. Essentially, each word has thousands of graded attributes, and, together, the numerical strength of these graded attributes encode that word's meaning. This is how LLMs turn language into a solvable math problem.

It would make intuitive sense to us to have clearly defined dimensions upon which each word is encoded, but that's not quite how LLMs work. You won't be able to see the numerical value for "maleness" and "royaltyness" for any given word. Instead, the dimensions used by the LLM do not have specific, explainable meaning to us, but when applied to the training dataset mathematically, they lead to similar words being represented with similar **embeddings** across these dimensions.

I know that was a bit technical, but this idea for how LLMs encode meaning is important for understanding how they work. Bear with me, as we have a few more technical details to get out of the way before we get to the more practical stuff.

## Tokens: The Currency of AI

To understand how LLMs read and write, you need to understand the concept of a token.

In the last section, I told you that models encode individual words. That wasn't entirely true. Models sometimes process whole words but also handle *parts* of words, and those words and parts of words can include punctuation. The unit of language that LLMs work in is called **tokens**. Why would they do this instead of dealing with whole words?

Let's think about a few words a model could encode:

- Thinking
- Processing
- Driving
- Susan's
- Joseph's
- Company's

In the first three examples, the "-ing" part of the word has the same meaning, and it relates to the first part of the verb stem. In the last three, the "-'s" indicates the possessive. If you were programming a computer, would it make the most sense to have separate embeddings for "think" and "thinking," or would it make more sense to have separate embeddings for "think-," "process-," and "driv-," plus one more for "-ing" since the "-ing" encodes the same thing for all three? Rather than having six different "words" encoded in the model, you can convey the same meaning with four tokens.

So, rather than encoding meaning for individual whole words, LLMs encode meaning in terms of tokens, which can either represent whole words or parts of words. A short word like "cat" might be one token, whereas "hypernatremia" might be broken into three.

Do you see where this is going? Breaking down hypernatremia into three tokens (hyper-natr-emia) allows us to more effectively encode the meaning of concepts like "hyperkalemia" and "hypophosphatemia" based on patterns we see in language. (A quick note: tokenization (breaking down words into their constituent tokens) is model-specific and not always linguistically clean—think "chunks of text" rather than true word stems. Different models will also split the same word differently.)

Current models include hundreds of thousands of distinct tokens in their vocabulary. If you're wondering how many "tokens" are in a sentence, a good rule of thumb is that the average token is about three-quarters the length of the average word. The average seven- or eight-word sentence will be made up of roughly ten tokens.

Why do I spend time talking about this nuance? It's because when you put a prompt into a model and get a response out, your usage is metered and charged by the token. More specifically, vendors typically charge per million tokens. The more tokens you put into the model—and the more it puts out—the more expensive your query becomes.

## The Context Window: Why the AI "Forgets"

This brings us to an important limitation of an LLM: the context window.

The **context window** is the model's "working memory." It is the maximum number of tokens the model can hold in its "brain" to process at any one moment.

Let's say a model has a context window of 8,000 tokens (about 6,000 words). If you paste a 10,000-word research paper into the chat box and ask for a summary, the model cannot process the entire document at once. This explains a phenomenon that frustrates many first-time users: the long chat thread.

Let's say you start a chat thread called "Grant Brainstorming." You talk to the AI model about your idea on Monday, you add some notes on Wednesday, and you ask it to help you write a draft on Friday. Every single time you send a new message in that chat, the software often takes the *entire history* of that conversation (or a rolling window of it, sometimes with earlier messages summarized) and sends it back to the model as part of the prompt as context. Because of this, each prompt in a chat becomes successively longer and longer. Because you are re-sending that lengthy history with every new message, long chats can become unexpectedly expensive and slow to process. The end-result is that long chats get slower, costlier, and can lose granular details.

When your conversation becomes so long that it exceeds the model's context window, one of two things happens. Either the oldest messages sequentially fall out of the context window (and the model completely forgets what you told it on Monday), or the system tries to quietly summarize and compress the older messages before continuing. This process goes by different terms, like **summarization** or **compaction**, depending on the vendor. The system condenses your earlier conversation into a shorter version to make room for new messages.

Compaction is a practical necessity, but it comes with real trade-offs. Think of services that provide high-level, brief summaries of books. The appeal of a 15-minute summary is that you get the key points without investing the six or twelve hours it would take to read the entire book. But anyone who has read both the summary and the original knows that something is lost in the summary—the supporting context, the nuance, the repetition that helps you remember, and the color that brings the author's argument to life. The summary is useful, but it is not the same as the book. The same is true when an AI system compacts your conversation: the model retains the broad strokes but loses the granular details you may have carefully provided. I'll share a concrete example of how compaction bit me in Chapter 11 when we discuss building custom AI skills.

This idea of summarization and context loss applies more broadly to how we use AI for information synthesis in our daily work. If you rely constantly on AI-generated summaries—of your inbox, your meeting notes, your journal articles—you are, by definition, losing some of the original context. The summary of a document is not the same as the original. This doesn't mean summaries aren't useful; they absolutely are. But it's important to recognize that when you outsource your reading to a summarization tool, you won't have all the context in your head, and you won't be able to incorporate that missing context into your thinking. Use summaries as a starting point, not a final destination.

**The guardrail:** Treat AI chats like disposable scratchpads. Do not keep a single chat going for three months. Keep your sessions focused on a specific task. When you move to a new task, start a fresh chat. If you have key facts the model must know, pin them to the top of your new prompt so they are fresh in the context window. For multistep tasks, consider creating one chat per step and using the output of the first step as the input for the second step, and so on.

## Key Takeaways

- An LLM is not a database of truth. It is a sophisticated autocomplete that predicts the next most probable token in a sequence based on patterns in human language.
- Words are encoded as vectors (embeddings) in multidimensional space, allowing the model to mathematically encode meaning and compute relationships between concepts.
- LLMs process language in units called tokens—not whole words—and usage is metered and charged by the token.
- The context window is the model's working memory. Long conversations become expensive and can lose details when older messages are summarized (compacted).
- Treat AI chats like disposable scratchpads. Start fresh conversations for new tasks, and keep key facts at the top of each prompt.

# Chapter 5: Control Knobs and the Reality of Hallucinations

Have you ever typed the exact same prompt into an AI model twice, but received two totally different answers? If the model is just a computer program, shouldn't it give you the exact same output every time, like a calculator?

It would, if it weren't for a few control knobs built into the software. The two most important ones are called "temperature" and "top-p." You don't need to know the math behind them; you just need to know what they do because they explain why you don't get the same output every time. Some call them the "creativity dials," and they explain a lot of the peculiar behaviors we see from LLMs.

## Temperature and Top-p (nucleus sampling)

Remember how we said the LLM calculates the statistical probability of the next word?

Let's say the model is trying to finish the sentence: *"The cat has pointy ..."*

If you look under the hood, the model might create something like the following probability table. (These numbers are illustrative—the real values would depend on the specific model and context, but the concept is the same.) The table shows, in order, the likelihood of each token coming next given the tokens that already exist and the order in which they appear in the sentence stem. Here, you see that "ears" is the most likely next word, predicted to come next 52% of the time. This is followed by "teeth," which happens 14% of the time, and so on:

| Rank | Token | Probability (p) | Cumulative p |
|---|---|---|---|
| 1 | ears | 0.52 | 0.52 |
| 2 | teeth | 0.14 | 0.66 |
| 3 | claws | 0.10 | 0.76 |
| 4 | ears. | 0.05 | 0.81 |
| 5 | whiskers | 0.05 | 0.86 |
| 6 | little | 0.04 | 0.90 |
| 7 | tail | 0.03 | 0.93 |
| 8 | paws | 0.03 | 0.96 |
| 9 | eyes | 0.02 | 0.98 |
| 10 | fangs | 0.01 | 0.99 |
| — | other tokens (combined) | 0.01 | 1.00 |

We'll discuss the "cumulative p" column in a bit, but for now, all you need to understand is that this is a ranked list and that the probability of each token coming next is listed in the "probability" column.

If the **temperature** is set to zero, the model will almost always pick the most probable token. There are some technical reasons (which I won't bore you with) why this behavior doesn't always hold true 100% of the time—but for all intents and purposes, think of a temperature of zero as meaning that the model acts strictly deterministically—it will *always* pick the most probable token. It will say "ears" (virtually) every time when given this prompt.

But if you turn the temperature up, you are telling the model to take risks. You are giving it permission to pick the less probable words. At a high temperature, it might occasionally say "teeth," or even "claws." The lower the temperature, the more monotonous and "safe" your responses will be. The higher the temperature, the more creative and "wild" your responses will be. Remember that an LLM predicts the next word based on the previous words, so adding a less probable word early in the sentence could take the ending of the sentence in a totally different direction.

If you are using a consumer-facing app, the temperature is usually hard-coded somewhere in the middle. The developers want the AI to sound natural and conversational, not like a robotic textbook. Later, when we look at advanced tools, you will try adjusting these dials yourself.

As a quick rule of thumb for temperature:

- If you are asking the AI model to brainstorm new research hypotheses or suggest creative titles for a presentation, you might want a *higher* temperature. You want it to connect disparate ideas and produce something more novel and creative.
- If you are asking the AI model to extract inclusion criteria from a clinical trial protocol, you probably want a *lower* temperature. You want zero creativity. You want strict, boring compliance.

**Top-p** (also referred to as **nucleus sampling**) refers to the probability distribution that the model will pull responses from. OK, what does that actually mean in English? If you look at the table in the last example, the "cumulative p" column sums the probabilities of the words in the list as you go from most likely to least.

When top-p is set to 0.9, the model ranks all possible next tokens by probability and works down the list, adding the probabilities until the cumulative probability hits 0.9. It then ignores everything that comes after that in the list. The result is a shortlist, and the model picks from that shortlist alone.

Using our above example, if the top-p is set at 0.9, then only the first six words on the list are fair game to use as the next token because *cumulative p* reaches 0.90 at token #6 (and would exceed it at #7). The list of options the model has to choose from becomes reduced to the following:

| **Rank** | **Token** | **Probability (p)** | **Cumulative p** |
|---|---|---|---|
| 1 | ears | 0.52 | 0.52 |
| 2 | teeth | 0.14 | 0.66 |
| 3 | claws | 0.10 | 0.76 |
| 4 | ears. | 0.05 | 0.81 |
| 5 | whiskers | 0.05 | 0.86 |
| 6 | little | 0.04 | 0.90 |

The concepts of temperature and top-p sound similar—and that's because they both work together, but they are fundamentally different. To summarize, top-p is a parameter that is set in the model to choose which set of words are options for the model to choose from (i.e., the "menu" of words to choose from). Temperature dictates how sharply the model favors the top choices versus considering less likely ones. The higher the temperature, the more often you'll see words from lower on the list.

## The Elephant in the Room: Hallucinations

Understanding the model as a mathematical probability engine performing the role of autocomplete with an adjustable "creativity dial" helps explain the most dangerous and inseparable flaw in generative AI: hallucinations. A **hallucination** is when the AI model confidently states a fact that is completely, undeniably false. It's when it "makes up" the answer.

When this happens, it is easy to anthropomorphize the AI model and accuse it of "lying." But these systems cannot lie because lying requires an intent to deceive and a fundamental understanding of what the truth is. The AI system doesn't *know* what truth is. It only knows what language looks like. For this reason, hallucinations are not a bug that can be entirely patched out. They are a fundamental feature of how the underlying math works. If we give these models the agency to be creative and conversational, we have to accept that sometimes their creativity will drift outside the boundaries of reality.

Does this mean we shouldn't use AI in healthcare? Absolutely not. It just dictates *how* we use it and the guardrails we should apply.

In the next chapter, we are going to look at a technology specifically designed to rein in these hallucinations and make AI safer. It's called Retrieval-Augmented Generation, or RAG for short, and it's about to become a major part of your daily workflow. You might already be using it and not even know it.

## Key Takeaways

- Temperature controls randomness: low temperature produces predictable, deterministic outputs; high temperature produces creative, varied outputs.
- Top-p (nucleus sampling) controls which tokens are available for the model to choose from by setting a cumulative probability threshold.
- These two parameters work together to shape model behavior—top-p defines the set of tokens the model can pick from next, and temperature dictates how often less frequent tokens are selected.
- Hallucinations are an inseparable flaw of LLMs. They occur because the model generates statistically plausible text, not verified truth.

# Chapter 6: RAG (Retrieval-Augmented Generation)

## AI Taking an "Open Book" Test

In the last chapter, we talked about hallucinations. The earliest publicly available LLMs answered medical questions like a medical student taking a closed-book exam, relying entirely on the language patterns they were exposed to in training and calculating the statistical probability of the next token, one token at a time. But what if, instead of a closed-book test, we let the model refer to outside resources? What if we let it take an *open-book* test?

That's exactly what newer models do. For complex prompts (or ones that need information published after the model finished training) the model can fetch outside content and ground its answer in that content. In the simplest example, it performs a web search based on your prompt, "reads" the top results, and bases its response on what those pages contain. More broadly, this technique of identifying relevant snippets from outside documents and injecting them into the model's context window so it can answer the question based on those snippets, is called **retrieval-augmented generation**, or **RAG** for short. Web search is one form of RAG; later in this chapter we'll see how the same idea works against a curated, pre-indexed corpus, like a hospital policy library.

It's as if we ran a PubMed search on a topic, handed the LLM a stack of peer-reviewed papers, and said: "Answer my question using ONLY the information in this stack of documents. And when you give me the answer, tell me exactly which page and paragraph you found it on." RAG is the single most important technical concept you need to understand if you are going to use AI for clinical decision-making. So many of the clinical AI tools you encounter from this point forward are likely to be built on it. As healthcare-specific foundation models continue to develop, some may encode domain knowledge directly without relying on RAG—but for now, RAG remains the dominant approach for grounding AI in authoritative clinical sources.

Prominent tools for medical professionals that rely on RAG today include OpenEvidence and UpToDate Expert AI. The former utilizes a collection of peer-reviewed manuscripts and guidelines as its "source of truth" and the latter uses the vast set of expert-curated UpToDate articles as its source of truth. By constraining the model to use a set of curated, discipline-specific, authoritative content, you significantly increase its accuracy on domain-specific tasks.

## How RAG Actually Works

Remember our discussion about embeddings from Chapter 4? We talked about how text is converted into mathematical vectors, plotting words like king, queen, prince, and princess in a multidimensional space based on attributes of what those words mean. This was how meanings of words were mathematically encoded in a way that the LLM can make sense of them.

RAG uses that exact same concept, but instead of encoding general knowledge, it indexes domain-specific knowledge so it can be retrieved and injected into the model's context at query time.

Let's say your hospital takes its entire library of clinical policies and runs them through an embedding model. Those policies are broken into smaller pieces ("chunks") and the meaning of those chunks is encoded into vectors (embedded). Think back to the king, queen, prince, princess example. These chunks of text are mathematically embedded so that similar concepts appear near each other in multidimensional space. This process is called **embedding**.

When you sit down at your computer and type the prompt, *"What is the hospital's protocol for administering high-dose methotrexate to a pediatric patient?"*, the system doesn't immediately send that question to the LLM.

Instead, it performs a two-step process:

**Retrieval:** The system takes your prompt and identifies which embedded chunks of the policies are closest to your question in multidimensional space. It retrieves the specific snippets from the policies that it identifies as potentially relevant to answering your question. These most relevant passages get pulled out and set aside.

**Augmented Generation:** The system then packages your original question plus those retrieved passages together and drops them all into the LLM's context window. It essentially says to the model: *"Here are snippets from the policy library that are most relevant to this question, and here is which policy each came from. Now, answer the question based on the information provided."*

## Why RAG Is a Game Changer (and How It Still Fails)

RAG dramatically reduces hallucinations. We call this **grounding**. Because the model is looking directly at the source text within its context window, it doesn't have to guess based on what it saw in the training dataset. It can answer based on ground-truth information from authoritative sources. It can also provide a citation linking right back to the original source where it found the answer so you can verify it directly.

But RAG is not flawless. If you understand how it works, you can easily predict its failure modes. First, the model is only as good as the documents it retrieves. If your hospital hasn't updated the referenced policy in years, the retrieval engine is going to fetch a stale, outdated document. The LLM will then generate a beautiful, confident, highly accurate summary of a potentially out-of-date policy.

Second, the retrieval step can sometimes just pull the wrong document. The system might retrieve the adult oncology policy instead of the pediatric one, or it might pull a guideline for a different disease altogether. The LLM will then synthesize the information from the guideline it retrieved, assuming it's what you wanted, even though it does not apply to your clinical situation.

RAG makes AI safer, but it does not remove your responsibility to verify. Always demand citations in your prompt and review them.

## Key Takeaways

- RAG lets the model take an "open-book test" by retrieving relevant documents and injecting them into the context window before generating a response.
- By grounding answers in authoritative sources, RAG dramatically reduces hallucinations and enables citation-backed responses.
- RAG is only as good as the documents it retrieves—outdated policies or incorrectly matched documents can produce confident-sounding but completely incorrect answers.
- Tools like OpenEvidence and UpToDate's Expert AI feature use RAG to ground clinical answers in curated medical literature.
- RAG makes AI safer, but it does not remove your responsibility to verify. Always demand citations and review them.

# Part III: Your AI Cockpit

# Chapter 7: My AI Tech Stack (and What Each Tool Does)

Now that you understand how the engine works, it's time to look at the cars we can get behind the wheel of.

Before I list specific tools, an important caveat: what follows is a non-exhaustive sampling of the tools I have gained personal familiarity with and the categories I think are most useful for clinicians today. There are many excellent tools I do not cover, and the AI landscape changes every week—the specific apps I mention here may look very different, be acquired, or be displaced by competitors by the time you read this. Do not get deeply attached to brand names. Get attached to the *function* each tool serves, and be ready to move to a different app if it better suits your needs or if another company's newest model becomes better than what's already out there.

## The Big Three: Generalist Chatbots

These are the heavy hitters. You access them through a web browser, a desktop app, or a mobile app. They are available as free versions, paid subscriptions, and on a pay-as-you-go basis through the Application Programming Interface (API).

- **ChatGPT (OpenAI):** Historically the most famous, ChatGPT has become the "Kleenex" of large language models. It has historically been a good all-around model. It doesn't have the usage limitations that Claude has, which makes users feel less constrained when using it. Some users find it more stale for writing tasks when compared to competitors, and there remain limits on deep research.

- **Claude (Anthropic):** Claude has gained popularity over the several months leading up to publication of this book. Some find that it has a more natural, less "robotic" writing style than competitors. Its "Projects" feature is a way to do personal RAG with your own files. Its usage limits remain a major pain point for users who are not willing to pay for the pricier subscription tiers.
- **Gemini (Google):** Gemini is deeply integrated into the Google ecosystem. If you use Gmail or Google Drive, Gemini can seamlessly pull context from your emails and documents. It can help you edit Google Docs directly within the document.

## How Subscriptions Work (and What You Get for Your Money)

Most people who use these tools on a day-to-day basis will use them through a subscription rather than paying per token through an API. The subscription model is simpler: you pay a flat monthly fee and get access to the models through the vendor's web, desktop or mobile app, often with some usage limits.

The pricing tiers are remarkably consistent across the Big Three. Generally, there are three levels. Broadly speaking, the **free tier** provides you with access to older, less capable lightweight models with more restrictive usage caps—enough to get a taste, but not enough to integrate AI into your daily workflow. The **standard paid tier** (roughly $20 per month) unlocks the vendor's current flagship model, higher usage limits, and extended access to "deep research," in addition to other features. The **premium tier** (roughly $100-$200 per month) provides you with access to the most capable models, the highest usage allowances, and "pro" features, like deep research features.

Two hundred dollars a month might sound steep—and for casual use, it probably is. But ask yourself: what is an hour of your time worth? Whether you measure that in clinical billing revenue, hours reclaimed from a grueling schedule, or simply time back with your family—if the tool saves you several hours per month, it has likely paid for itself. That said, most clinicians will find that the $20 per month tier provides more than enough capability to meaningfully improve their workflows. You don't have to break the bank to use some of the best AI models.

## The Aggregator: OpenRouter

If you want to try out a dozen different frontier models without buying a dozen subscriptions, you can load a few dollars into an OpenRouter account and access all the major models on a pay-as-you-go basis. You can also pit models head-to-head using the same prompt and see the different responses each provides. This is the tool we'll be using in Chapter 8 when we roll up our sleeves.

## The Privacy Tool: Ollama

What if you have a document that is sensitive, and you don't trust vendors to process it, even if they claim they do not train using your data? Or maybe you are in a place where you don't have internet access, like on an airplane that hasn't yet been updated with Wi-Fi. You can use **Ollama**. Ollama is a free program that allows you to download smaller **open-weight models**—models which are publicly available for anyone to download and run on their computer or mobile device. These are "mini" versions of models that are small enough to fit on your computer and run on your hardware. The trade-off with using these models is that because they have to be small enough to fit on your computer, they aren't quite as capable as the cloud-based frontier models. If you download a bigger model and try to run it, you'll see that it runs much slower than you're used to when you're interacting with the model on the cloud. This is because your computer simply doesn't have the same processing power that the servers powering popular LLMs have. If nothing else, this experience will demonstrate just how compute-intensive these models are.

If you're looking for the local model experience on a mobile device, several apps are available, including Apollo and Edge Gallery.

## LLM-Powered Search: Perplexity

Think of Perplexity as an AI search engine. Give it a prompt, and it will turn it into a search, feed the top search results to a foundation model (e.g., ChatGPT, Claude, Gemini), and provide the answer to your question, grounded in those results. It works remarkably quickly and has fairly generous usage allowances. Its "deep research" feature doesn't crawl the internet as deeply as the analogous features provided by the Big Three and is subject to usage limitations, but Perplexity is a good go-to for quick, direct answers grounded in up-to-date information from the internet. Crucially, it provides direct links to the sources it used so you can quickly verify its claims.

## Voice, Dictation, and Transcription

As busy clinicians, typing often slows us down. We can usually talk faster than we can type. Real-time transcription models are becoming increasingly used to allow you to speak instead of typing.

- **On-device Transcription:** The built-in dictation on modern smartphones has become highly accurate with on-device AI. In many languages, speech is converted to text without the data leaving your device.
- **Superwhisper:** This is an AI-powered dictation app that runs on your computer or mobile device. It is privacy-focused and allows you to run part or all of the pipeline using locally run models (similar to how Ollama works) so that your data never leaves your computer unless you allow it to. It works in two steps: using one speech-to-text dictation model to transcribe your speech into text, and then using a general-purpose LLM to clean and format it. You can incorporate specific prompts for different scenarios to customize the output (e.g., format as a formal business email) so that what you say is processed and formatted differently for different use cases.

## Audio Consumption: ElevenLabs / ElevenReader

I am a huge fan of audiobooks. The only times I can seem to find to read are when I'm driving in the car or doing chores around the house. In the rare case when I actually have time to sit down and read a book, I often don't have the mental capacity to read off the page. Listening is just so much easier. But you can't buy an audiobook version of the latest journal preprint article or a draft manuscript you're writing and want to review one more time. This is where realistic text-to-speech services come in. The Big Three all have versions of this, but for my money, none performs as well as ElevenLabs.

- **ElevenLabs / ElevenReader:** ElevenLabs uses incredibly lifelike, AI-generated text-to-speech. I first encountered their models when listening to audio versions of *The New Yorker* magazine and was amazed by how lifelike they were. I can point it to a website, paste text or upload a file, and ElevenReader will add the text to my account and read it aloud in a natural, conversational voice of my choosing. As I iteratively refined this book, I used ElevenReader to listen to early drafts. Hearing the text read aloud revealed awkward phrasing and structural issues that I skimmed over when reading silently. The text-to-speech algorithm sometimes injects stray sounds or awkward inflections, but I find these easily forgivable given the convenience it provides. One of my favorite use-cases is having a general-purpose LLM generate a detailed Deep Research report on a topic, then export that report for listening using Elevenreader. ElevenLabs provides access to a variety of other fun generative AI tools, including image, video, and music generation.

## RAG for Medical Knowledge

- **UpToDate Expert AI:** UpToDate's RAG-based tool grounds AI-generated answers in UpToDate's extensive library of curated medical content.
- **OpenEvidence:** This RAG-based tool grounds AI-generated answers in peer-reviewed medical literature and guide-

lines published by major professional societies. When I first used OpenEvidence, I worried that the answers it gives might not be as practical, since its knowledge base focused on the medical literature rather than expert-curated encyclopedic articles like those found on UpToDate. However, I have been pleasantly surprised by how well OpenEvidence practically applies its knowledge base to patient cases.

- **ChatGPT for Clinicians:** Brand new as of the time of this writing, this is OpenAI's tool that serves a similar function, grounding answers in the published medical literature. It also includes functionality to assist with writing patient-facing materials.

## Ambient Transcription and Note Writing

- **Ambient scribe:** Examples include DAX Copilot, Abridge, Ambience and Suki. The concept is simple: the system listens to the visit, transcribes the conversation between you and the patient, and then uses that information to draft your note. There are many ambient scribing products on the market—so many that they are quickly becoming a commodity.

Documentation burden is consistently one of the top drivers of physician dissatisfaction, so it's not surprising that these tools have been rapidly adopted over the past couple of years. Overall, I've found these tools to be a major productivity booster compared to typing notes or even using speech-to-text software. They also make for a more pleasing patient encounter where you can focus on being present in the conversation, rather than furiously jotting down notes.

The strengths and limitations I describe here are broadly representative of the category because they are all based on similar models working under the hood. These systems generally perform very well at capturing the patient history, but in my experience, performance is underwhelming for writing the assessment and plan. In large part, this may not represent a fatal flaw in the system itself, but rather in the way that it captures information about the plan. We often don't describe our medical decision-making in as detailed of terms when conversing with patients as we do when we document in our notes.

I also find the current model's note-writing style to be stiff, and it doesn't capture my personal "voice". While the inner workings of these tools are not completely transparent for proprietary reasons, this default "voice" is most likely due to tuning and/or prompting that the vendor has built into the model. I have found that significant improvements can be gained by adjusting the system prompts that are run immediately before generating the final note, yet there is still much left to be desired. My hope is that future iterations of these tools will be able to be trained on historical notes that an author wrote to capture their voice.

If, like me, you find the ambient listening feature to be underwhelming for capturing the assessment and plan, here's a trick: you can dictate the assessment, medical decision-making, and plan to the tool after the visit to ensure your thought process is captured in the note.

## Let's Roll Up Our Sleeves

Hearing this list might feel overwhelming, but remember this: you don't need to use all of these. I'm just sharing some examples of tools that I use so you can check them out and use the ones that fit best in your workflows. You don't have to dive in and use them all at once. Feel free to try them out one at a time, or just try out the ones that you think you would use most. In the next section, I'm going to show you a quick and inexpensive way to test-drive and compare models from the major AI labs, from the "Big Three" and beyond. This allows you to see how the "top-tier" models compare to the older "lower-tier" models. You can compare output styles of different models and see how prompt engineering can influence the responses, while playing with parameters like top-p and temperature to see how they affect the outputs.

Are you ready? In the next chapter, we'll log into OpenRouter, spend five dollars, and put everything you've learned so far into practice. Let's go!

## Key Takeaways

- The Big Three consumer chatbots (ChatGPT, Claude, Gemini) each have distinct strengths and weaknesses; try several to find which tool or tools best suit you.
- Open-weight models allow you to process sensitive data locally without it ever leaving your device, at the cost of reduced capability.
- Dictation tools, text-to-speech services, and ambient scribes are rapidly maturing and may reduce documentation burden.
- Don't get attached to brand names—the tools will change. Get attached to the *function* each tool serves and be ready to switch when it suits you.
- You don't need to use all of these tools. Start with one or two that fit your workflow and expand from there.

# Chapter 8: The OpenRouter $5 Lab

Up to this point, we have been talking about AI in the abstract. Now, it's time to get our hands dirty. In the opening chapter, I told you that you should use AI early, often, and on a variety of tasks. We're now ready to dive in and do just that.

If you've been stuck using a free version of an AI tool, I'm going to ask you to do yourself a favor. I'm asking you to take $5 of your hard-earned cash and use it to play with some of the newest and most capable AI models. I recognize that it might seem silly. You might ask, "Why would I pay $5 for something I can get for free?" Please, just trust me. It's a low-stakes way that you can see the differences between these models firsthand.

We're going to be using a tool called OpenRouter. To give you some context for how it works, I need to explain a concept called an API. You probably thought the technical part of the book was over. Please—stick with me! This one's pretty quick, and I'll try to explain it with a relatable analogy that you'll understand.

## Application Programming Interfaces

**API** stands for **Application Programming Interface**. It sounds like computer science jargon, but you likely actually use APIs every day without even knowing it. APIs are simply the ways that computers and computer programs talk to one another behind the scenes.

Think about how you book a flight for a medical conference. You don't go to Delta's website, write down their flight options and prices in a notebook, then go to United's website, and then go to

American's website to do the same. Maybe you use an aggregator like Google Travel or Expedia, or perhaps your employer requires you to use a platform like Concur. In these tools, you type in your local airport, the destination airport, and when you want to travel, and the website magically shows you all the flights from all the airlines in one neat list.

How do these sites work? Perhaps you imagine that each day, they download each airline's flight schedule and pricing information and store it in a database that they reference when you run your query. There are a few reasons why this approach isn't practical. First, daily downloads fail to give you up-to-the-minute availability information, which is important when it's possible someone just bought the last available seat, yet the website is still showing it for sale. Second, it is inefficient to download every possible routing combination and fare—point-to-point between any two airports in the world—across the entire calendar year daily for every airline.

Instead, these services use APIs. Think of an API as a digital messenger. The aggregator sends a digital message to each airline (or a vendor that serves data from the airline) and says, "What flights do you have on September 1st from Fargo to Chicago?" The message is sent in a pre-specified format that the recipient knows to expect. Pre-specified "rules of the road" dictate the minimum necessary information that must be sent with a request (e.g., date of travel, origin, destination, and number of passengers) as well as other optional parameters (e.g., preferred class of service). Delta's computer then sends a message back with the flight options (i.e., flight numbers, times, and price) in a predictable, computer-readable format that the aggregator can then put into a user-readable, branded format alongside results from other airlines. These systems work quickly—that's why it's possible for the system to do an instantaneous search and return the results in just a couple of beats.

AI systems also run on APIs. Sure, you can use the web browser interface for ChatGPT, and that works just fine. But what if you are a company that is continuously putting out content, and you want to automate your use of LLMs? Let's say you're a newspaper, and you want AI to generate three "what you should know" bullet points for every article you publish, and put them at the top of the article. You could make the writer paste their article into ChatGPT, ask it to give high-level bullet points, and include them when they submit the article to the editor. Alternatively, your publishing software could automatically send a copy of each story along with a pre-filled prompt (i.e., "Summarize the article into three 'What you should know' bullet points. These should be concise and written at a fifth-grade reading level.") to an LLM API, which will automatically return the summary to the publishing software in real time, putting that summary alongside the full article automatically.

In short: APIs are the connectors that let AI scale beyond a single person typing into a chat box. They make it possible to embed model output directly into the software, workflows, and tools we use every day. For the rest of this chapter, we're going to use APIs ourselves to take a few of the major models for a test drive on a pay-as-you-go basis.

## Creating an OpenRouter Account

For this exercise, we'll use OpenRouter to interact with a variety of large language models through their APIs. OpenRouter is one of several pay-as-you-go AI aggregators. I'm using OpenRouter here because the user interface is approachable for non-technical users and OpenRouter provides access to a wide variety of models. That said, you don't have to use OpenRouter; if you prefer another aggregator, feel free to follow along using whichever one suits you.

Go to **openrouter.ai** and click the blue "Sign up" button in the top right to create an account. Then click the hamburger menu (three horizontal lines) in the top right and select **Credits**. Add $5, and—importantly—**disable "auto top-up"** so additional credits aren't charged to your card without your knowledge.

Now we're ready to explore.

## Exploring the Models

Click on "Models" on the top menu. As of the day I'm writing this, OpenRouter had 657 models available for use. You're probably thinking, "How in the world do I choose between all of these?!"

On the left-hand side, you'll see a filtering menu that allows you to narrow down the models to just the ones you want. Let me explain some of these options.

- **Input modalities:** This tells you what types of input prompts you can give the model. Will it accept text only? Can you attach files to add context? Can you add images for it to analyze?
- **Output modalities:** What will it output? Will it generate text *and* images? Can it narrate the output as audio?
- **Context length:** As we discussed earlier, the context length (also referred to as the context window) refers to the model's working memory. How many words (more precisely, how many *tokens*) can it hold in its working memory to answer your questions?

- **Prompt pricing:** OpenRouter allows you to filter between free, inexpensive, and expensive models. We'll dive more into the specifics of this in a little bit.
- **Series:** These are the different "brands" of models.
- **Categories:** These are suggestions for things that the model is felt to be "good" at. Some models are better at computer programming, others are better at drafting scientific documents, and others are better at writing ad copy. It's not that one model is inherently *better* than another. Each was simply trained differently, and that training becomes reflected in the model's outputs. The result is that each model has relative strengths and weaknesses depending on the task it's being asked to complete.
- **Supported parameters:** This section includes some terms that should now be familiar to you, like temperature and top-p. This allows you to filter by models that let you tweak these parameters, which we'll be playing around with in Chapter 9.
- **Zero Data Retention (ZDR):** When ZDR is enabled, your input is used solely to process your request and generate a response; it is not logged or stored on the vendor's servers afterward, and it's not used to train the vendor's models. This is important for privacy-sensitive uses.
- **Providers:** These are the different cloud companies that actually run the models on physical computer servers. You might assume that if you want to use ChatGPT, you'd click "OpenAI" here, but that's not how it works. Under Providers, click "Amazon Bedrock," for example. Here, you will see some models by Amazon, but you also see models by other AI labs, like Anthropic and OpenAI. One of OpenRouter's claims to fame is that for a given model, it may have several providers it can route your request to. The

same AI system is running in different places, giving you redundancy in case a specific server is down or running slowly.

- **Model authors:** The AI lab that developed the model. Here, you'll see names like Anthropic, OpenAI, and Google. This list is probably longer than you thought it'd be, filled with many companies you've never heard of before. This is the landscape of AI today, and this is why I wanted to bring you here to OpenRouter: to see what's out there.

## Individual Model Pages

Now, let's pick a model. You can pick any one you want. Click on the model name on the main part of the page, or search for one you've heard of. For this example, I'll search for GPT-4.1 and select **OpenAI: GPT-4.1**. OpenRouter shows you a little leaderboard on the right-hand side with how many billions of tokens OpenRouter passed to that model in the past week. You'll see some tags for things that model is described to be "good" at, a narrative description about the model, the context window size (in thousands or millions of tokens), the price per million input and output tokens. If you click on the specific model name, you'll see the model page, where you can see which different cloud providers the model is available through. The Benchmarks section shows you how well the model performed on a variety of benchmark tasks.

I have assembled a very crude summary table listing some of the popular models you might see on OpenRouter with pricing as of this writing in April 2026. **A word of caution: model names, pricing, and availability change frequently. Treat the names and prices below as illustrative snapshots, not definitive. Veri-**

**fy current information at openrouter.ai/models.** The comparisons here are not based on quantitative comparisons, so you should treat them as incomplete and oversimplified summaries designed to orient the beginner. My goal here is to introduce you to some of the models I'm familiar with, and to help you build a mental model for how to choose which model to use for which task.

| Model | Producer | Local / Cloud | Speed | USD per 1M input tokens | USD per 1M output tokens | Best For |
|---|---|---|---|---|---|---|
| **Claude Opus 4.6** | Anthropic | Cloud | Slow | $2.01 | $25.00 | Critical thinking, research, and complex analysis requiring deep judgment |
| **Claude Sonnet 4.6** | Anthropic | Cloud | Fast | $1.13 | $15.00 | Best quality/speed/cost balance in the Claude line; "daily driver" |
| **Claude Haiku 4.5** | Anthropic | Cloud | Very Fast | $0.60 | $5.00 | "Easy," lightweight tasks that require rapid responses |

| | | | | | | |
|---|---|---|---|---|---|---|
| **GPT-5.4 Pro** | OpenAI | Cloud | Slow | $30.00 | $180.00 | Highest-stakes tasks where cost is secondary; critical reasoning |
| **GPT-5.4** | OpenAI | Cloud | Moderate | $2.35 | $15.07 | Strong general-purpose model |
| **GPT-5.4 Mini** | OpenAI | Cloud | Very Fast | $0.21 | $4.49 | "Easy," lightweight tasks that require rapid responses |
| **Gemini 3.1 Pro** | Google | Cloud | Slow | $1.16 | $12.03 | Demanding critical reasoning, long-document synthesis (thanks to large context window) |

| | | | | | | |
|---|---|---|---|---|---|---|
| **Gemini 3 Flash** | Google | Cloud | Fast | $0.32 | $3.00 | Everyday development and asks where cost and speed matter more than quality |
| **Gemma 3 27B** | Google | Local + Cloud | Fast | $0.10 | $0.29 | Privacy-sensitive local deployments; offline or air-gapped environments |
| **DeepSeek V3.2** | DeepSeek | Local + Cloud | Fast | $0.21 | $0.48 | Value frontier model; general tasks, reasoning |
| **DeepSeek R1** | DeepSeek | Local + Cloud | Slow | $0.70 | $2.53 | Step-by-step reasoning |

| | | | | | | |
|---|---|---|---|---|---|---|
| **Qwen 3.6 Plus** | Alibaba/ Qwen | Local + Cloud | Fast | $0.00 | $0.00 | Reasoning model competitive with the "Big Three" frontier models |
| **Qwen 3.5 Plus** | Alibaba/ Qwen | Local + Cloud | Fast | $0.41 | $2.40 | Everyday general tasks at low cost |
| **Qwen 3.5 Flash** | Alibaba/ Qwen | Local + Cloud | Very Fast | $0.10 | $0.40 | High-volume, speed-sensitive workloads where cost must be minimized |

*Source: openrouter.ai model pages, April 2026. Pricing reflects weighted average. Pricing changes frequently. Speed indicators are crude generalizations, not quantitative comparisons. Verify and get up-to-date model pricing at openrouter.ai/models*

Let's break down a few things as we review this table. First, I need to be clear that the "speed" categorizations are relative generalizations, not quantitative comparisons. And when I say a model is "slow," I don't necessarily mean it is going to take an eternity to get a response—its speed is just slow *relative* to the other, faster models.

While the "Big Three" have a variety of models, you'll find that the offerings of major vendors tend to reflect a general pattern that I'll summarize:

- "Fast and cheap": a very fast model that is inexpensive to use at high volumes. The trade-off is that these models are not as capable as the slower, more expensive models. These are often used by developers needing to have an LLM perform a relatively straightforward task where speed and cost are paramount.
- "Daily driver": this is the "Goldilocks" model; capable enough for most everyday tasks, yet not cost-prohibitive to operate. These models are often the main offering of free tiers. It's often the case that last year's flagship model becomes this year's daily driver.
- "Flagship model": this model performs best on reasoning tasks and is used when the quality of the output trumps cost and speed concerns. This is what "power users" will be using much of the time. You might need to be on a paid tier to use these models.

As we discussed in Chapter 7, Ollama and similar tools allow you to download **open-weight models** and run them locally on your computer, meaning your data and the responses you receive never leave your environment. This makes them worth serious consideration for anyone working with sensitive or proprietary information. If your hardware isn't up to the task of running a large model at a usable speed, you can also deploy these same models on a cloud server. These models often cost a fraction of what comparable "closed-weight" models cost to use.

Some of the most capable open-weight models currently available, including DeepSeek and Qwen, are developed outside the United States. Running them locally keeps your data on your own device, but the model weights themselves originate abroad, which can matter for regulated workflows. Before incorporating any open-weight model into a regulated project—such as one governed by federal research data requirements or export controls—check whether the model's provenance is compatible with your funder's, your organization's, and the government's policies on supply chain risk.

## So, How Much Is This Actually Going to Cost Me?

### Pricing of a Versatile Model

Let's go back to our previous example prompt. I'm going to enter this prompt into GPT-4.1 and see what comes out:

**Me:** The cat has pointy ...

**GPT-4.1:**

It looks like your sentence is incomplete. Would you like to finish it, or are you looking for examples of how it might be completed?

Here are a few possibilities:

The cat has pointy ears.

The cat has pointy teeth.

The cat has pointy claws.

The cat has pointy whiskers (though usually we say "long" whiskers).

If you want a specific continuation or more examples, let me know!

Using the OpenAI Tokenizer—an app that shows you how many tokens a piece of content contains—I can see that my query used 6 input tokens. The output was 87 tokens. Based on an input price of $2 per million tokens and an output price of $8 per million tokens, that query cost me $0.000708. I would have to run that prompt 15 times to use up a penny of my credits.

## Pricing of a "Premium" Frontier Model

Let's see how different models compare. GPT-5.4 Pro is OpenAI's most capable model as of the time of this writing. For prompts less than 272,000 tokens, the input price is $30 per million input tokens and $180 per million output tokens.

Compared to GPT-4.1's $2 per million input tokens, GPT-5.4 Pro charges 15 times as much, and for output tokens, it's over 22 times as expensive.

Let's run our example prompt using GPT-5.4 Pro and see what happens.

> **Me:** The cat has pointy ...
>
> **GPT-5.4 Pro:**
>
> *Reasoning: Considering sentence completion*
>
> *It seems like the user is looking for a way to complete the fragment "The cat has pointy...". My guess is they want to fill in the blank with something like "ears" since it's a natural fit. However, they might be looking for something rhyming too? Given that their input was minimal, I'll just respond simply with "ears." This keeps it concise without overcomplicating things or needing any math.*
>
> ears.

The first thing you might notice is that GPT-5.4 Pro is taking longer than GPT-4.1. That's because it's "thinking" (we discussed earlier that these models aren't capable of cognition, hence the quotes). The model is *emulating* thinking. This extra "thinking" is why we're paying big money for our input and output tokens. There's also this "reasoning" box, where the model is explaining its "reasoning," walking us through its thought process. It then gives a simple, one-word (two-token) output answer: ears.

You might be thinking, well, this isn't so bad. I'm paying $180 per million output tokens, but the output was only two tokens. Not so fast—those "reasoning" tokens also count against your output token price. So we actually are paying for more like 93 output tokens.

If we do the math, how much did that prompt cost me? $0.017—nearly two cents. The cost of this query isn't preventing me from paying my mortgage, but two cents seems a bit steep to understand which body part on a cat is pointy!

This illustrates the trade-off of using a highly capable model versus a lightweight and inexpensive model. The more expensive models can provide higher-quality outputs, but they aren't needed for simple tasks. The same query cost 24 times more with GPT-5.4 Pro, and I basically got the same answer.

Now you've encountered the first cost limitation: model price. While GPT-5.4 Pro is available to anyone with API access on a pay-per-use basis, only users on OpenAI's $200/month subscription tier can access it through the website and app. Those on the $20/month tier are constrained to GPT-5.3 in the web interface.

The total cost is also dependent upon the number of input and output tokens. This is where things can easily get out of hand. My example prompt didn't use that many tokens, but let's consider a few examples.

1. You ask an LLM to search PubMed for case reports on a rare patient presentation. It goes out, searches the web, reviews all of those case reports in their entirety, and then reports back based on those results.
2. You give a hospital-approved LLM all of your hospital policies and ask it to identify all instances of redundant or contradictory policies.

3. You ask the LLM to ingest a transcript of a four-hour meeting and generate a summary.

In the first example—the web search—every word on every page the LLM processes counts against your input tokens. I recently asked Claude to identify as many pediatric oncology chemotherapy regimens as possible and to compile a structured list to serve as a chemotherapy regimen "library." On one query, it reviewed and analyzed nearly a thousand webpages, with each token from each website counting as an input token.

Earlier, we discussed how context is important—the more relevant context you provide the model with, the more relevant its output will be. This, too, comes at a cost. All of that context costs you in input tokens. If you upload a copy of your CV when you ask the model to write a cover letter for a job you're applying for, you're paying for the model to process every token within your CV.

The last cost factor I'll discuss is chat length. We discussed earlier how the context window—the size of the LLM's working memory—can be a limitation. For this reason, it's a best practice to create a new chat for each topic or subject. There's another reason it will benefit you to create new chats: each time you send a message, the entire chat history is fed back into the model as input tokens for context. While input tokens are generally cheaper than output tokens, it is important to understand that in a long chat, each query becomes successively pricier in terms of input tokens. Some models get around this limitation by periodically summarizing ("compacting") the conversation; in essence, the LLM creates a concise summary of the conversation thus far and then uses that (instead of the original conversation verbatim) as the input context. This is helpful for two reasons: first, it allows you to overcome limits of model context windows;

second, it saves money on input tokens. The drawback is that each time the LLM summarizes, some of the richness of the original conversation gets lost in summarization.

In OpenRouter, you can choose how many of the previous messages are included in each prompt you pass to the LLM, allowing you to manually balance the extent of context with the cost of additional input tokens.

## Exercise 1: The Side-by-Side Comparison

Before we continue, I need to explain a small difference between how the OpenRouter APIs and your traditional LLM interface work. Remember when I talked about Zero Data Retention? If a provider commits to process your data and then delete it, how do you look back at your old chats? You certainly can't go back to that provider to ask for them because they don't have your data anymore.

Unlike consumer chatbots that save your chats in your account and let you access them from any computer, OpenRouter's chat tool stores your queries and the LLM responses locally in your browser once they are returned. Because these are not stored on OpenRouter's servers, chat history will not sync across browsers and devices. If you clear your browser's memory store, you will lose all of these chats forever.

Let's do a little head-to-head experiment. In your OpenRouter account, click on Chat from the top menu.

Now, click "New Chat," then Add Model. Click Input and select "text" since we'll be entering text queries to start. You can pick any model on the list—it really doesn't matter which one—then add two more models by clicking the "+" icon. For example, you can select OpenAI GPT-5.4, Claude Opus 4.6, and Gemma 3 27B. The first two models are flagship models from large vendors, and Gemma 3 27B is a free, open-weight model that you can download and run on your computer if you wanted to (or you can run it off a cloud server, as we're doing here). Enter a prompt. I'm going to prompt with a clinical-administrative scenario:

> **Me:** I am a pediatric oncologist. Draft a letter of medical necessity to an insurance company appealing a denial for dordaviprone for diffuse midline glioma. Be professional, firm, and concise.

Hit enter.

Now, analyze two things: the speed at which each model generates the output, and the substance and style of the output.

The first thing you'll notice is the speed difference I highlighted in the table above. While the frontier models excel at complex tasks, the trade-off is speed. For most people typing into a chatbot and reading the response, the speed difference is inconsequential because one can only read so fast. But consider how this calculus might change if you are using an LLM to perform real-time voice interactions on a customer support phone call—the speed becomes much more important to ensure the conversation flows smoothly.

Another difference you'll probably notice is the richness of the response. Less capable models tend to write in a more generic, slightly robotic tone and might be prone to hallucinate more. In contrast, the frontier models will write you a highly nuanced, persuasive letter. They will likely use appropriate terminology, cite sound rationale, and strike a tone that sounds like a confident and experienced physician.

Finally, are you starting to get a feel that each model has a unique "style"? Beyond how lifelike and accurate the output is, some models might have a more friendly, casual, and conversational style. Others may be more succinct, matter-of-fact, and professional. These differences reflect both the data that the models were trained on and how the model's "control knobs" (like temperature and top-p) are set. I highlight this difference to point out that which model is "best" is not strictly about performance on a standardized test. "Best" is in some respects subjective and dependent upon the task you're trying to perform—you want to match the right worker for the task they're best suited to perform.

The differences you see in model outputs are what I was trying to explain at the beginning of the book when I suggested that you don't want to "drive last year's car." Some LLMs are better than others, and in my opinion, the better ones are worth spending money on.

## Exercise 2: Model Switching

Another cool thing you can do with OpenRouter is change models mid-chat. Remember how we discussed that recent chat history is sent along as context with each query? Because recent messages are re-sent each time—regardless of which model generated them—it doesn't matter which LLM produced the previous response. The new model picks up the thread seamlessly.

Create a new chat using any model and start talking. Then, click the X on the model name (to remove that model) and add a different model. Keep chatting. See how the chat doesn't miss a beat?

Going back to our example of when to use the expensive models versus the inexpensive ones, switching can be an efficient way to use models: use the expensive models for the difficult "cognitive" tasks, and use the inexpensive ones for the simple ones, like proofreading and information retrieval.

As I mentioned earlier, OpenRouter allows you to adjust how many recent messages get sent along with each request (see the chat bubble icon with a number next to it—the default is usually 8). Try tuning this down to one or two and have a conversation with the model. After a while, ask it about something that happened earlier in the chat. Did it remember?

Now that you've seen how to compare models head-to-head and switch between them mid-conversation, let's go deeper. In the next chapter, we'll twist those "creativity dials" we discussed in Chapter 5—temperature and top-p—and see exactly how they shape the model's output. We'll also try our hand at generating images.

## Key Takeaways

- OpenRouter is an aggregator that lets you access hundreds of AI models on a pay-per-use basis without committing to individual monthly subscriptions.
- AI model pricing varies enormously: lightweight models can cost fractions of a penny per query, while premium frontier models can cost anywhere from several cents to several dollars.
- The pattern across vendors is consistent: "fast and cheap" models for simple tasks, "daily driver" models for everyday use, and "flagship" models for complex tasks.
- You can switch models mid-conversation in OpenRouter because recent chat history is re-sent with each query, regardless of which model generated it.

# Chapter 9: Twisting the Dials—Temperature, Nucleus Sampling, and Image Generation

In the last chapter, we set up our OpenRouter account, explored the model landscape, and ran our first side-by-side comparisons. Now it's time to pop open the hood and play with the control knobs that shape how these models behave.

## Exercise 3: It's Getting Hot in Here—Twisting the Creativity Dials

Choose a model—any model—and click the three dots to the right of the model name. Notice a few things: the "enable reasoning" toggle (if the model offers "reasoning") will allow you to turn "reasoning" mode on or off. This allows the AI model to emulate thinking, which generally gives better results, but at the expense of more tokens. Now, look at the System Prompt. These are some default instructions that are provided to the model with every prompt. You don't see these in the chat window, but they are counting as input tokens that you get charged for in the background. These system prompts are yet another way the model can be fine-tuned for specific scenarios. The system prompt box tells you how many tokens it is costing you to include this system prompt.

Now let's get to the fun part. Click Sampling parameters. These are the knobs under the hood you can play around with. Don't worry, you won't break anything here.

The first one is **max tokens**—this tells the model the maximum number of tokens it can return as the output. I find that the models are generally pretty good at self-modulating, but if you're working with a model with high output token cost, you could consider constraining this. Decreasing this value can prevent queries from becoming expensive, but at the cost of having less detailed responses.

Next, we have **temperature**. Think of this as the "spiciness" and variability of the model's outputs. Let's be extreme—turn the temperature all the way down to 0. Now, enter a prompt. I entered a boring prompt:

**Me:** Create a poem about a rock.

**GPT-4.1:**

A rock sits still
and does not ask
for praise, or names,
or softer tasks.
It keeps the rain,
remembers heat,
lets moss and shadow
at its edges meet.
Once it was fire,
or mountain bone,
now it is patient,
small, and alone.
Yet in its silence
worlds pass through—
wind, hoof, river,
morning dew.
I hold it once.
It says no word.
Still, something ancient
feels quietly heard.

Not bad. Now, let's add some spice. Go back to the temperature setting and crank it all the way up to 2.0. So as not to bias the spicier version of our model with the initial boring version of the poem, create a new chat. Type the same prompt.

**Me:** Create a poem about a rock.

**GPT-4.1:**

A rock sleeps
where the hill forgets its name,
holding the sun
in a language older than fire.
Rain comes to read it,
wind comes to smooth
its rough gray thinking,
and moss writes green silence
across its back.
It does not hurry.
It does not ask.
It keeps the weight of centuries
like a secret in its bones.
And still, beneath the patient sky,
it shines—
not because it moves,
but because it remains.

Can you tell the difference? The first example was very predictable and literal. The second is more metaphorical and literary. This is the impact of temperature on the output.

Let's play with **top-p** now. Remember, this is the set of word probabilities that the model can choose from, and then temperature is the "randomness" with which tokens within that set are selected (versus always deterministically selecting the single most likely).

Keeping the temperature cranked up to 2.0, set top-p to 0.1 (very restrictive). Create a new chat and repeat the prompt. Here's what I got:

**Me:** Create a poem about a rock.

**GPT-4.1:**

A rock sits still
while days run past.
Rain writes on it,
wind hums low,
sun warms its back
with golden hands.
It does not hurry,
does not speak,
yet keeps the shape
of time.
Small and silent,
gray and plain,
it holds the mountain's
memory
in its sleep.

You've probably observed that the effect of changing top-p isn't as dramatic as changing the temperature, but the change in top-p affects the spontaneity of the output.

Just to review here, what's happening under the hood is this: when the model is attempting to predict the next token, it generates a list of possible next tokens along with a probability (between 0 and 1) of each token coming next in the sequence given the provided tokens.

Let's go back to the example of our pointy friends:

> **Me:** The cat has pointy...

Earlier, I showed you this example table, which is what an LLM might be considering for next-word possibilities. Probability (p) refers to the likelihood that a given token would come next. Cumulative p sums the p of a given word and all the words that came before it in rank order until you've accounted for all the word possibilities and cumulative p reaches 1.

| Rank | Token | Probability (p) | Cumulative p |
|---|---|---|---|
| 1 | ears | 0.52 | 0.52 |
| 2 | teeth | 0.14 | 0.66 |
| 3 | claws | 0.10 | 0.76 |
| 4 | ears. | 0.05 | 0.81 |
| 5 | whiskers | 0.05 | 0.86 |
| 6 | little | 0.04 | 0.90 |
| 7 | tail | 0.03 | 0.93 |
| 8 | paws | 0.03 | 0.96 |
| 9 | eyes | 0.02 | 0.98 |
| 10 | fangs | 0.01 | 0.99 |
| — | other tokens (combined) | 0.01 | 1.00 |

If you select a top-p of 0.9, that means that the model will restrict its output to only those tokens in order until the cumulative p reaches 0.9. In this case, any of the first six words are fair game when we have the top-p set at 0.9, but all the words from number 7 onward will be ignored as options. Next, the temperature dictates how often the model strays from choosing the most likely tokens to choosing less likely ones. Pick a temperature of 0, and you will get a response from the model of "ears" all the time (or nearly all the time). Pick a temperature of 2, and you'll be more likely to see "whiskers" and "little" creeping into your responses, though "ears" will remain the most frequent because its probability (p) is higher.

Take a careful look at items 1 and 4. The first is "ears" (without a period) and the fourth is "ears." (with a period). Aren't these the same thing? Not really—remember, we're dealing in units of "tokens" here, not words. To the model, "ears" (without a period) and "ears." (with a period) have different meanings, and that makes some sense. The token "ears." (with a period) finishes the sentence—it completes the thought. The token "ears" (without a period) still leaves open the possibility of either appending a "." to complete the thought, or continuing the sentence.

We might see an illustrative next-token probability table after "ears" (without a period) that looks something like this:

| Rank | Token | Probability (p) | Cumulative p |
|---|---|---|---|
| 1 | . | 0.42 | 0.42 |
| 2 | and | 0.18 | 0.60 |
| 3 | that | 0.10 | 0.70 |
| 4 | , | 0.08 | 0.78 |
| 5 | with | 0.07 | 0.85 |
| 6 | which | 0.05 | 0.90 |
| 7 | sticking | 0.03 | 0.93 |
| 8 | perked | 0.03 | 0.96 |
| 9 | twitching | 0.02 | 0.98 |
| 10 | like | 0.01 | 0.99 |
| — | other tokens | 0.01 | 1.00 |

Statistically, the most probable outcome is a period to end the sentence, but depending on the top-p selected, other tokens will be available, and the temperature setting will determine how often lower-probability tokens that continue the sentence (rather than terminating it) will come next.

Think of this process happening over and over again for every token in the response. That's precisely what's going on inside the LLM: given what was entered as the prompt and what has already been written, what is likely to come after that? You can see how a small change at the beginning of the response can have a dramatic impact on later tokens. A small change in the second token can change the most likely third token, which will then impact the most likely fourth token; and so on.

Let's do one more example before moving along. In our original prompt, replace "cat" with the plural form, "cats."

**Me:** The cats have pointy...

The LLM might generate an illustrative probability table like this:

| Rank | Token | Probability (p) | Cumulative p |
|---|---|---|---|
| 1 | ears | 0.48 | 0.48 |
| 2 | teeth | 0.15 | 0.63 |
| 3 | claws | 0.11 | 0.74 |
| 4 | noses | 0.07 | 0.81 |
| 5 | whiskers | 0.06 | 0.87 |
| 6 | tails | 0.04 | 0.91 |
| 7 | faces | 0.03 | 0.94 |
| 8 | paws | 0.02 | 0.96 |
| 9 | heads | 0.02 | 0.98 |
| 10 | features | 0.01 | 0.99 |
| — | other tokens | 0.01 | 1.00 |

We see some familiar players here—"ears," "teeth," and "claws" still dominate the most likely next words, but now the sleeper token "noses" creeps in and "tails" is now the sixth ranked instead of the seventh. Importantly, the token "ears." (with a period) is nowhere to be found here. By not including tokens that end with a period, the model is saying, in this case, "after this word, keep the sentence going." Linguistically, it might make sense that, given this prompt, the reader might expect more context about the pointy body part, rather than terminating the sentence.

Seeing this behavior demystifies the inner workings of AI. It reminds you that an LLM isn't a magical brain; it's a math engine that predicts the next token in a sentence based on patterns seen in human language. It is a highly sophisticated autocomplete.

The model's advanced settings include several other sampling parameters you can modify. We won't dwell on these here, but I'd encourage you to play around with them yourself. If you hover your mouse over each parameter name, OpenRouter will give you a brief description of what that knob does. Twist the dial and see what happens! Remember, you won't break anything here—I promise.

## Exercise 4: A Quick Note on Images

Before we leave the lab, let's try our hand at generating images using generative AI. Many of the platforms allow you to generate images from text.

Create a new chat, click the X on the last model (or models) you had loaded to clear all of the models, then click the + sign to add a model. Search for Nano Banana 2—this is an image-generating model from Google. In the text entry box, click "Create artifact" and click Image so that the output of the prompt is an image.

Try the prompt (or substitute your specialty):

**Me:** Image of a pediatric oncologist.

**Nano Banana 2:**

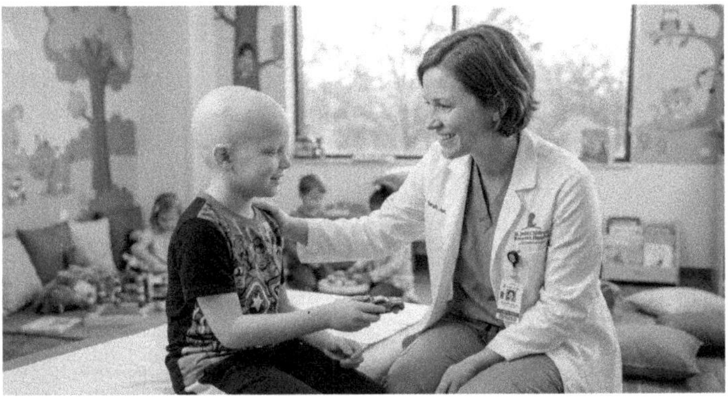

Let's break this down—there's a white, female doctor sitting across from a bald child. The doctor is wearing a white coat with a hospital logo and name that seem eerily similar to a well-publicized children's hospital based in Tennessee. The name on the doctor's lab coat appears to be a woman's name. The setting is a bit interesting: is this an exam room (as judged by the exam table), a playroom in the clinic, or some weird amalgam? And who are the kids in the background—are they other patients? Siblings?

If you look carefully, you'll notice that there are letters underneath the hospital name on the doctor's lab coat, but when you zoom in, things fall apart. They have shapes that are similar to letters, but aren't letters that exist in the English alphabet.

What you're seeing is that these models often present a blended "average" or an amalgam of what might be expected in a specific scenario, which often yields odd results.

You may also notice that before the image was generated, the model added some color to your admittedly boring prompt. This is the context the model added before generating the image:

> **Nano Banana 2:** Here is a natural portrait of a compassionate pediatric oncologist interacting with a young patient.

This is the model helping itself out. Before attempting to generate the image, it generates richer, descriptive text to give the image model some guidance. It is parlaying a large language model's ability to add color and imaginative description into a better result from the image model. You can do this yourself to have more control over the image composition—use any general-purpose LLM to help you think of and compose a scene and output a specific, detailed prompt for an image model.

Now, if we don't like this image, we can fix it up. Let's ask it to make a change:

**Me:** Make the doctor male.

**Nano Banana 2:**

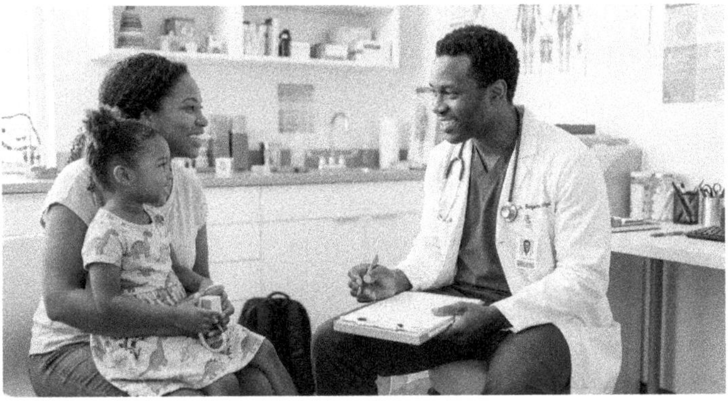

Quite a different result. Here, it didn't just put a male in the female doctor's place, but the scene is entirely different. It's a different room, different patient, and now a female caregiver is present with the patient.

Now let's have a little more fun. I uploaded a picture of me along with the following prompt and asked it to make a photo of me as a doctor.

**Me:** Make a photo of this person as a doctor.

**Nano Banana 2:**

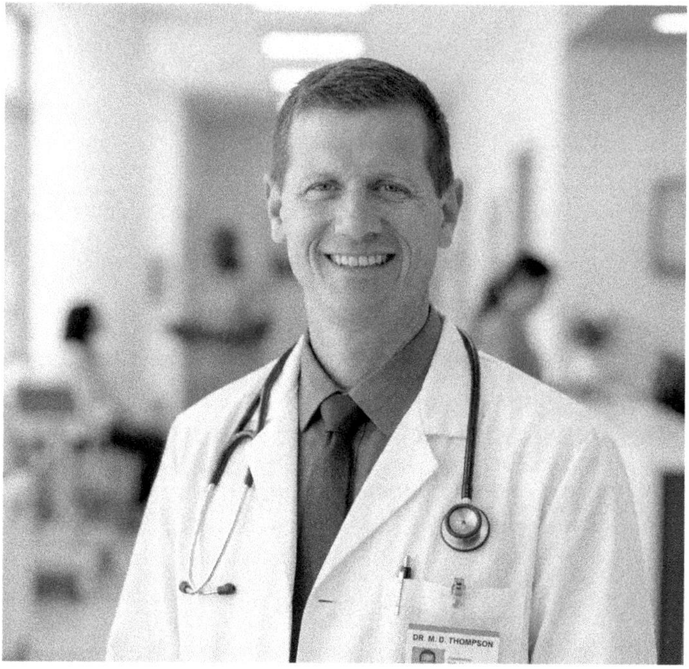


This looks identical to me. Now, let's put this character into action.

**Me:** Show that doctor as a pediatric oncologist holding a patient's hand while they receive an infusion.

**Nano Banana 2:**

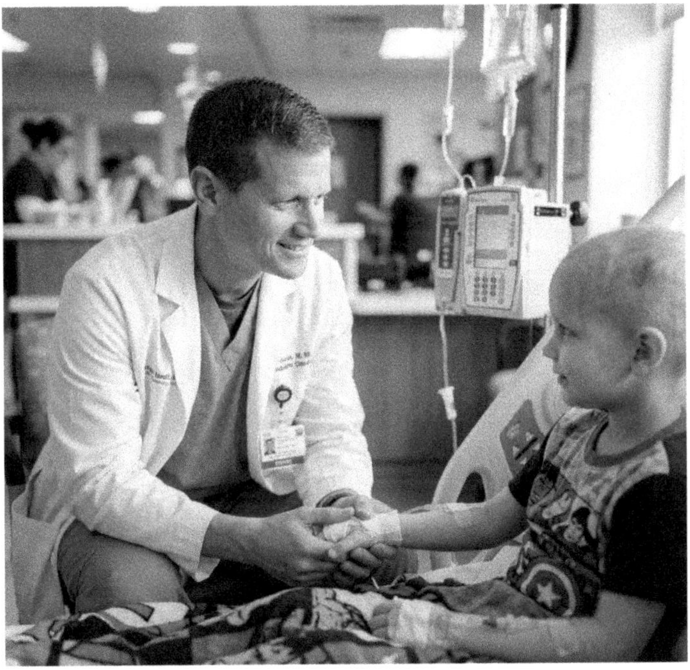

Impressive, right?

Let's try one last thing before we move on. Create a new chat and type these two prompts:

**Me:** Chest X-ray with right lower lobe pneumonia.

**Nano Banana 2:**

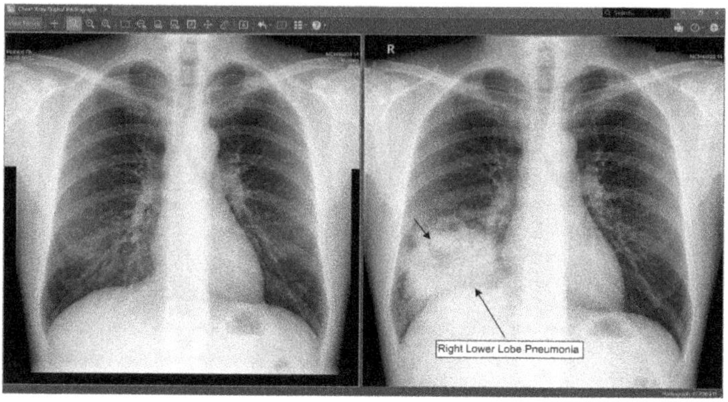


**Me:** Create a chest X-ray with metastatic osteosarcoma.

**Nano Banana 2:**

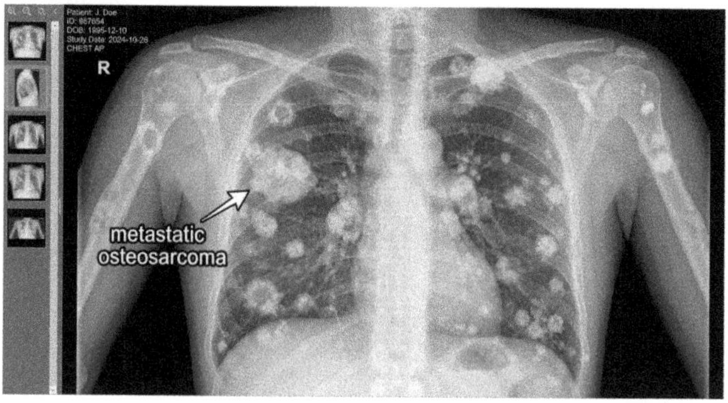

**Important:** Synthetic medical images are for demonstration purposes only. They contain artifacts and inaccuracies. Do not use AI-generated medical images for clinical diagnosis, treatment decisions, medical education, or training.

## So, What Did This All Cost You?

Before we move on from our OpenRouter experiment, let's do one last thing. Let's see how much this little adventure cost you.

Put your mouse over the "hamburger" (three horizontal lines) menu on the top-right and click on Credits. Click View Usage. Here you can see how many requests you made, how many tokens those requests consumed, and how much money they cost, all broken down by model. Notice how the price you paid for those images is two orders of magnitude larger than what you paid for your text queries? Image generation is *much* pricier than text generation.

I didn't walk you through video generation, but as a frame of reference to understand how much video generation costs, consider this: as of this writing, some generation models charge roughly $0.50 per second of video generated at full resolution. That means that a brief 10-second video costs $5 to generate! And I thought my two-cent query about which body part on the cat was pointy was expensive!

## Key Takeaways

- Experimenting with temperature and top-p firsthand reveals how these parameters shape output creativity and variability.
- Image generation models produce blended "averages" of expected scenes and often struggle with fine details like text and logos.
- You can iteratively refine AI-generated images through follow-up prompts, but each iteration may change the entire scene.
- Image generation is significantly pricier per query than text generation; video generation is more expensive still.
- Synthetic medical images are for demonstration only—never use them for clinical diagnosis, medical education or training.

# Chapter 10: Everyday Accelerators

Alright, you've survived the theory, the privacy warnings, and even my $5 OpenRouter experiment. You understand the engine, and you know how to drive. Now, let's actually go somewhere.

In this chapter, I'm going to give you some of my favorite "Everyday Accelerators." These are low-risk, high-return prompts that you can use on the proverbial "Monday morning" to instantly reclaim time.

## 1. The Email Polish

We all write emails or draft notes when we are rushed, or maybe just exhausted. We struggle to figure out how to clearly and concisely convey what we want to say. You could ask the LLM to "improve this," and it will probably improve your draft. But I'd ask you to resist this urge and, instead, be very specific and explicit about *how* you want it to be edited. Be as specific as possible about what you want from the model.

Consider a prompt like this:

> **Me:** These are rough thoughts I'd like to convey to my boss. Re-draft the email, fix the typos and grammar, and organize it into a logical flow with paragraph breaks. Crucially: I want to strike a relatable and empathic, yet firm tone. Do not add any corporate jargon.

And let's give the model an email like this:

> **Me:** Dr. Stevenson—I'm really frustrated by the new rollout of our new paging system. This happened with very little training and the rollout was so hasty and rushed, and we're all paying the price because people are having a difficult time getting ahold of other people. Nurses are upset at me. I have no idea how to contact a given patient's nurse, and the tech support line is unhelpful—all they do is tell me they'll "put in a ticket." I don't need a TICKET, I need a system that allows me to safely communicate!

I tried my prompt along with my original email as context using Claude Opus 4.6. Here's what I got back:

**Opus 4.6:**

Dr. Stevenson,

I want to share some concerns about the new paging system rollout, because it's creating real problems for patient care.

The transition happened quickly, with very little training, and we're now seeing the consequences. I'm struggling to figure out how to contact a given patient's nurse, and I know I'm not alone—nurses are frustrated too, and that tension is affecting all of us.

When I've reached out to tech support, the response has been that they'll "put in a ticket." I understand they have processes to follow, but what we need right now isn't a ticket—it's a reliable way to communicate safely with each other so we can do our jobs.

I'd appreciate any guidance you can offer, or the chance to discuss how we might address this more urgently.

Thank you,

[Your name]

Pretty diplomatic, right? It filtered out your anger and tried to keep things matter-of-fact, yet sensible and in a way that your boss would be more likely to respond to and wouldn't get you fired. But you think it's too polite and passive-aggressive—you're facing a serious problem, and your boss needs direct communication to understand just how urgent the situation is.

Let's view this as an opportunity to steer the model in the direction we were trying to go, even though that's not where it went at first:

**Me:** Be more direct about the consequences so that it stirs the boss to act and revert to the old paging system.

**Opus 4.6:**

Dr. Stevenson,

I need to raise an urgent concern about the new paging system rollout.

The transition happened quickly, with very little training, and we're now facing serious consequences. I cannot reliably reach a given patient's nurse, and nurses can't reliably reach me. This isn't just frustrating—it's a patient safety issue. When communication breaks down, critical information gets delayed or lost, and that puts patients at risk.

The tension is building among staff. Nurses are upset, I'm upset, and none of us have the tools we need to do our jobs safely. When I've called tech support, all I get is a promise to "put in a ticket." That's not good enough when we're talking about patient care.

I'm asking that we revert to the old paging system until proper training is in place and the new system is actually ready for clinical use. The old system wasn't perfect, but it worked. What we have now does not.

I'm happy to discuss this further, but I don't think we can afford to wait.

Thank you,

[Your name]

I tend to prefer the "voice" of certain models over others—not because one is objectively better than the others, but because the voice more closely matches my personal language style and the tone I am trying to convey. Try a few models from different series and see which ones most closely align with your preferred style.

## 2. Rhetorical Tuning: "Imply This"

Sometimes, you know exactly what the facts are, but you are struggling with the right way to say it. You know that the words on the page—when read literally—say one thing, but when people read them, you worry they're going to hear something else. There's what the words say, and there's what people read between the lines. It's that latter part that you're struggling with. What if people get the wrong connotation? Similar to the last example, there are often ways that a sentence can be subtly reworded that entirely change the meaning and how others interpret it.

Let's give an example from a clinic note: "The patient has been poorly adherent to their oral iron."

Ugh, this sounds really judgmental.

> **Me:** Rewrite this statement to clearly communicate that the patient is not adherent, but state it in a way that does not imply negative judgment: "The patient has been poorly adherent to their oral iron."

Here, the model gives me several options to choose from, along with the connotations that correspond with each, and leaves it up to me to choose the one that fits best.

**Opus 4.6:**

**Original statement**

> The patient has been poorly adherent to their oral iron.

Below are several alternatives that communicate the same fact while avoiding negative judgment.

**Neutral clinical documentation**

> The patient has not been taking the prescribed oral iron consistently.

**Slightly more patient-centered framing**

> The patient reports difficulty taking the oral iron consistently.

**Barrier-focused framing**

> The patient has had difficulty maintaining consistent use of the prescribed oral iron.

**Objective chart language**

> Oral iron has been taken inconsistently.

**Collaborative tone**

> The patient has not yet been able to take the oral iron regularly as prescribed.

**Pattern illustrated**

> The rhetorical shift generally involves removing the subject-blame framing ("poorly adherent") and replacing it with neutral, process-focused language.
>
> The factual signal remains intact—**the medication is not being taken regularly**—but the language avoids implying blame or moral judgment.

## 3. From Meeting Transcripts to Action Items

If you have an administrative role, you probably sit in endless meetings. If your hospital allows recording and transcribing via an approved tool that meets your organization's security and privacy standards, an AI model can summarize it in seconds. This allows you to focus on the conversation rather than taking notes, and it ensures you don't miss important points.

If you use a note-taking system with configurable prompts, don't just ask it to "summarize this meeting." Be specific about what you want from it and what you want the output to look like:

> Attached is the transcript from this week's tumor board. Summarize each case as follows: 1. Patient initials and case ID (include only what is needed for the task), 2. Concise, four-sentence case summary, 3. Clinical question for the tumor board, 4. Perspectives and opinions (with attributions for who said what), 5. Final clinical conclusion, 6. Next action items and individuals responsible.

**Important:** Because this transcript likely contains PHI—patient names, dates of birth, and/or identifiable clinical details—this task should only be performed using a HIPAA-compliant, BAA-covered AI tool approved by your institution. Do not use a personal or consumer-grade AI account for tasks that include protected health information.

## 4. The RFP/Grant Crosswalk

Applying for grants or responding to Requests for Proposals (RFPs) is a notoriously tedious process of matching your past work to their specific requirements. You've got lots of great skills and ideas to build off your past work, and the funding body that puts out the RFP has its own priorities. Where do those intersect?

Give the system the RFP and your most recent CV.

> Attached is my current academic CV (including past research) and the RFP for a new grant opportunity. Act as a research strategist. Draw parallels between the grant's requirements and my past publications and projects. Tell me which of my past work makes me a strong candidate, and identify the gaps in my experience that I need to address in my application narrative.

You can take this a step further by sharing nascent ideas you've been thinking about:

> I'm also interested in exploring the use of natural language processing to extract late-effects data from survivorship clinic notes. Tell me how this idea might align with the RFP's priorities, and what gaps in my previous work I would need to address to make this use case compelling.

## 5. Explain a Complex Concept in Lay-Friendly Terms

As clinicians, we suffer from the "curse of knowledge." We know our subspecialties so deeply that we forget what it is like to *not* know what "neutropenia" or "intrathecal" means.

When you're trying to summarize a complex concept in patient-friendly terms, have the model give you ideas for how to more clearly explain it.

> Here is a draft of a handout I wrote for families about an upcoming chemotherapy regimen. Read this from the perspective of an anxious, exhausted parent with a 6th-grade reading level who has just spent three days in the hospital. What parts of this handout are confusing, overwhelming, or needlessly full of medical jargon? Give me specific suggestions to make it more empathic and easier to understand. Use understandable analogies when possible.

**Note:** Your institution may require that patient education materials go through a formal review and approval process before distribution. While AI can be a helpful tool for drafting and refining these materials, be sure to follow your organization's policies and procedures before sharing any written education materials with patients.

## Making AI Useful, Right Now

These five accelerators we just discussed don't require you to be a computer programmer. They just require you to view AI as an extremely fast, highly literal assistant sitting next to you at your desk.

In the next chapter, we are going to push the boundaries a bit further and look at some more advanced workflows—like building your own personal AI prompt library and giving the AI model a memory. Strap in—we're about to put the pedal to the metal.

## Key Takeaways: The Accelerators

- The Email Polish: Edit emails for clarity when you're having a hard time organizing your thoughts into a concise and coherent message.
- Rhetorical Tuning: explore how subtle rewording can subtly modify the meaning of your message and the way others read between the lines.
- From Meeting Transcripts to Action Items: Provide transcripts with a structured output template to extract decisions, attributions, and next steps.
- The RFP/Grant Crosswalk: Upload your CV alongside an RFP and your research priorities to identify areas of alignment and gaps that need to be addressed.
- Explain a Complex Concept in Lay-Friendly Terms: Re-craft your message with jargon removed and concepts explained in terms anyone can understand.

# Chapter 11: Advanced Workflows—Where the Real Leverage Hides

The "Everyday Accelerators" we just covered are great for quick wins. But if you want to fundamentally change how much work you can get done in a day, you have to move beyond typing simple, individual questions into a chat box.

You need to build systems and advanced workflows. You need to make the AI model sweat. This is where the real leverage hides, and where the "super-users" are separated from the "basic" users. This is what will set you apart so that you remain competitive in a world full of AI tools.

## 1. Working with Files and "Lightweight RAG"

Modern LLMs don't just process text you type; they can process files you upload and ground their answers in the content of those files. You can drag and drop PDFs, Excel spreadsheets, and Word documents directly into the chat window. In addition to reading files, they can also create files. You can give a model a PowerPoint template and ask it to put together 15 slides following an outline you provide while maintaining the style used in the template

We reviewed earlier how important it is to give the LLM as much context as possible. By attaching files to your prompts, you can create a personal version of the RAG system we talked about in Chapter 6.

For example, Anthropic's Claude has a feature called "Projects," and OpenAI has "Custom GPTs." These features allow you to upload a stack of specific documents—say, your division's entire fellowship curriculum, call rules, and vacation policies—and save them into a dedicated workspace. You are instructing the model, *"Whenever I chat in this specific Project, use these uploaded documents as your source of truth."*

If you instruct the model:

> A first-year fellow wants to take vacation during the second week of their inpatient oncology block. According to our rules, is this allowed, and who needs to approve it?

The AI model will retrieve the applicable rules from your PDFs and give you an answer grounded in those rules.

## 2. The Personal Prompt Library (and Custom Skills)

Once you realize how powerful a well-engineered prompt is (remember our Role, Task, Context, Constraints, and Format framework from Chapter 2?), you will quickly realize that you do not want to retype that giant paragraph every time you need it.

Do not rely on your memory. Build a **prompt library**. Think of these as your "dot phrases" for the LLM—the prompts you use over and over again and that work really well for you in predictable, repeatable situations.

The prompt library doesn't have to be anything sophisticated. It can be a simple Word document or a note on your phone. Personally, I use a Google Document with multiple tabs that I can access from anywhere.

Let me give you an example of how this can be useful.

When I submit a grant application, I want to be sure that it's polished and ready to submit. We need to ensure that all abbreviations are spelled out at their first mention, that the table and figure numbers are sequential, and that my colleague's preference for Oxford commas is applied—that every "and" at the end of a list has a comma before it. We want to identify typos or major grammatical errors and ensure that we aren't missing any of the content or formatting requirements listed in the request for proposals. This is not the time to critique the research aims for scientific validity and flag the proposal for a complete rewrite, but rather to make sure we're ready to submit and haven't overlooked any details. I'm not asking AI to write the grant for me; I'm asking it to proofread.

For tasks like this, you can create reusable prompts that specify exactly what you're looking to double-check. You can even upload a copy of the RFP for the model to reference to ensure you are meeting all of the explicit requirements. In this way, you can build the tool once and use it countless times.

## From Prompt Library to Custom Skills

If you want to take this concept even further, the major AI platforms now offer features that let you save and reuse your most refined prompts as persistent, reusable tools. OpenAI rolls them into their "Custom GPTs" feature. Anthropic calls them "Skills" and also rolls them into its "Projects" feature. The names differ, but the concept is the same: you create a detailed set of instructions that gets automatically injected into every conversation in that workspace.

Here's the thing that surprises most people when they peek behind the curtain: these "skills" are not sophisticated software. They are not apps built by engineers. Instead, they are nothing more than carefully written and refined prompts. They are a structured, specific, and explicit set of instructions for how to perform a given task, saved in a way that the model can reference them, and the model uses them every time you start a new chat.

Let that sink in for a moment, because it reveals something profound about just how powerful careful prompting really is as a skill. The five-component framework we discussed in Chapter 2—Role, Task, Context, Constraints, and Format—is the exact same framework that powers these "skills." The difference between a casual prompt and a polished skill isn't a difference in the underlying technology; it's a difference in the level of detail, specificity, and refinement you put into the instructions. A Custom GPT or skill is just a prompt that has been tested and refined through iteration until it reliably does what you want.

This is why I spent so much time on prompt engineering earlier in this book. When you learn to write a great prompt, you aren't just learning to have a better one-off conversation with an AI model. You're learning to build tools that work exactly how you want them to. You're developing the ability to create reusable, reliable workflows that you can invoke with a click, share with colleagues, and refine over time. The prompt is what makes the tool yours. The same model is available to everyone, but the way you prompt it is what sets you apart from the average user who has access to the same tools.

The process of building a skill is straightforward: you tell the model what to do, what not to do, and what the output should look like. You run it. You look at the result. You tweak the instructions if you're not getting exactly what you want. You run it again. Over several iterations, you converge on something that works reliably. Every time the model strays from what you want, you go back to the prompt and add a more specific instruction—often a negative constraint—that closes off the unwanted behavior. It's a virtuous cycle: each failure teaches you how to write a better prompt for that model, and each better prompt produces a more reliable skill. Yes, this takes some time and patience—and in today's fast-paced world you might feel like you don't have the time or patience to "train" your LLM—you want it fully trained out-of-the-box. But this is what I mean when I talk about using LLMs *collaboratively*. Don't have the LLM do your work for you—that's lazy. Leverage the LLM's capabilities, along with your knowledge and cognitive effort, to build something truly remarkable. **That's where the magic is.**

Let me give you a real example from my own life. At our house, we have about 25 standby meals that we rotate through. These are meals that we know are easy to make, that use ingredients we typically have around the house, and that everyone in the family likes. Every week, we need to plan what meals we're going to have. This is often dictated by our schedule, and it's something I would rather not have to invest a lot of time and energy in. If I'm on call one night, we need a meal that's easy for my wife to prepare on her own. If I'm working from home, or it's a weekend, slow-cooker meals are great—we throw the ingredients together midday and dinner is ready by evening. If we're taking our kids to T-ball practice right after work, it's peanut butter and jelly sandwiches that we'll pack and eat at the practice field right before practice starts. And if I've got a full day at home without a lot going on, I might want to cook something on my pellet grill.

I asked Claude to help me develop a skill that would handle this meal planning. The idea was that the skill would know which meals my family likes to make and understand the constraints around when we might want to make each one. For example, I'm the only one in my family who grills. My wife likes to make slow-cooker meals over the weekend when I'm on call. I like to grill in the summer, but not in the winter. The skill would take a general idea of our schedule for the week and produce a meal plan that follows specific rules, like not repeating the same meal twice in one week.

It took about an hour of back-and-forth with the model, but I was able to refine this skill until it worked exactly how I wanted it to. Now, this skill lives inside my set of Claude skills as a carefully crafted prompt that gets injected whenever I ask it to plan our meals for the week. I give it a rough outline of our schedule, and it gives me a meal plan that actually makes sense for our family.

Here's what I want you to take away from this example: everything I just described—the meal constraints, the schedule logic, the rules about not repeating meals—lives inside a text prompt. That's it. No computer coding. No database. Just a really detailed, really specific set of instructions written in plain English. **The barrier to building your own AI tools (and using AI in general) is not technical expertise; it's the willingness to be specific about what you want and to iterate until you get it right. Careful, deliberate, and thoughtful prompt engineering is the number-one skill you can develop as an LLM user.**

## When Compaction Bites: A Cautionary Tale

Remember when we discussed compaction in Chapter 4—how long conversations eventually get summarized to save space in the context window? Here's where that concept became very real for me.

When I was building my meal planning skill, I provided links and PDFs to all of those recipes at the very beginning of the chat. Once I got the meal planning logic working the way I wanted, I had a thought: wouldn't it be great if the model could also generate a grocery list for the week based on the meals it planned? I figured this would be straightforward since I had already given the model all the recipes.

But between the time I originally provided those recipes and the time I asked for the grocery list feature, the conversation had gotten quite long with all of the back and forth, and the model compacted it. When that happened, the links to the recipes all disappeared from the context window. The model remembered that a recipe existed and that I had provided a link to it, but it didn't know what the link actually was because the link was removed during the compaction process. It needed me to provide those links again, which created extra work I wasn't expecting.

This is the book summary problem in action. The compacted summary preserved the gist—"user has recipes for these meals"—but it lost the specific details I needed. It's a good reminder that compaction preserves the broad strokes but drops the granular details, and you should plan accordingly. For important reference material, keep it in a persistent location (like a Project or a Custom GPT's knowledge base) rather than relying on it surviving a long chat thread.

### 3. AI "Memory"

Many models incorporate a "Memory" feature. Across all your different chats, the AI model will quietly take notes on things you tell it—like your preferences and major events (e.g., you're going on a vacation to France in June, you're applying for a new role at work). If you mention in one chat that you are a pediatric oncologist in North Dakota, and in another chat that you prefer bullet points over paragraphs, the AI model can remember this and ground its responses in this context.

Under the hood, this "memory" is really just a sophisticated version of the system prompt we discussed in Chapter 9. The model distills facts about you over time as you chat with it into a concise summary, which is then automatically injected into every new conversation as a hidden prompt. This is worth pausing on, because it reinforces just how central prompting is to nearly everything LLMs do—just like the last two "advanced workflows," this one's just another prompt that gets injected into your conversations.

Memory can be incredibly helpful. You no longer have to explain who you are every time you log in, and the AI model learns how to tailor its responses to you—just like a helpful personal assistant who has worked with you for years.

But it can also be a liability. Sometimes the model remembers things you *don't* want it to apply universally. Maybe you asked it for advice on how to handle a delicate personal situation, and then the model brings up that personal situation in a cover letter you're writing for a promotion. Or, it relies more heavily on this context than you want it to (e.g., it knows you are a pediatric oncologist, and when you ask it to help you draft a letter of interest for joining your local school's parent-teacher association, it emphasizes your role as a physician over your role as a parent).

**The guardrail:** Go into your AI model's settings and look at its Memory block. Most providers have a way to update this so that you can delete things you don't want it to remember and add things you do. Alternatively, you can turn the feature off entirely if you prefer a blank slate for every new chat.

## 4. Connectors and Agents

We are entering an era where AI doesn't just sit in a chat box; it connects directly to your other apps—sometimes through traditional APIs (which we talked about in Chapter 8) and increasingly through newer standards like the Model Context Protocol (MCP), which provides a standardized way for AI models to discover and use external tools and data sources. Implementation details may differ slightly between providers, but the practical concept is the same: the AI model reaches out to another system, reads and/or writes data, and incorporates the result into its response. When you grant an AI model access to your email account, it can summarize your inbox, identify high-priority emails needing your attention, and take a first stab at drafting a response.

This enables **agentic** behavior—meaning the AI acts as an "agent" performing tasks on your behalf. You can say:

> Look at my calendar for next week, find a 45-minute gap, and draft an email to Dr. Smith proposing times when we could meet to discuss the new leukemia trial.

The AI model will read your calendar, suggest a time, and draft a response to Dr. Smith.

This can be powerful, but it also creates risk. Connectors introduce significant data leakage risks. We are going to cover the security implications of this in Chapter 12, but for now, know that connecting an AI model to your inbox should be done with extreme caution. Your business email and calendar accounts should only be connected to an AI system if approved by your employer and with appropriate security measures in place.

## 5. "Vibe Coding"

As a clinical informatician, I'd say I'm more knowledgeable than the average person when it comes to computer coding. But my coding days were long ago, and those skills are rusty. Fortunately, you don't need to know a single programming language to use AI to make computer programs that do whatever you want. You can build websites and apps that do just about anything. This type of coding by non-coders using natural-language prompts that describe what the code should do is termed **vibe coding**.

It's worth pausing to appreciate the implications of LLMs writing code. When you ask an LLM to summarize a paper or draft a patient education handout, it's producing English-language prose. A remarkably powerful capability of modern LLMs is that they can also write in the language of computer code. And code isn't just text—it's a set of instructions that a computer can actually execute. When the LLM writes code, that code can do things:

crunch numbers, pull data from other software, generate visualizations, automate workflows, even build entire applications from scratch. This is the difference between an LLM telling you how to solve a problem and an LLM just solving the problem itself.

Let me give you an example of just how powerful this feature is. "Roadmaps" are a staple in pediatric oncology. They are a communication tool that clearly presents a chemotherapy regimen in an easy-to-understand graphical and tabular format. In less than an hour, I was able to ask Claude Opus 4.6 to (1) gather pediatric oncology chemotherapy regimens from the internet (it searched nearly 1,000 webpages), (2) integrate them into a website that allows users to view graphical representations of the regimen, (3) create a calendar of what chemotherapy will be administered on which day when a start date is specified (and export to someone's existing digital calendar), and (4) export a Word document with the roadmap. I was able to create this as a locally run web app on my computer after providing iterative feedback to the LLM about improvements I'd like to see from earlier versions. Now, the app wasn't perfect, and there were some nuances about the chemotherapy regimens it didn't pick up on. It definitely wasn't production-ready, but it was surprising how it got far more things right (without any explicit direction) than it got things wrong.

Just as when you use connectors, there are risks with vibe coding. If you don't know how to read and understand what the code says—what the code is doing—how can you be so sure it is safe to run on your computer?

## 6. Deep Research and Web-Grounded Search

One of the most powerful capabilities the Big Three platforms now offer is the ability for AI models to autonomously search the web, read dozens or even thousands of pages, and synthesize the findings into a structured report. This capability goes by different names depending on the platform—usually called something like "deep research"—but the core concept is the same: instead of answering your question from memory alone, the model actively goes out, searches the web, places what it finds in the context window, and grounds its response in those sources.

This is a significant step forward from standard chat-based interactions, and it offers two key advantages.

First, because the model is grounding its answers in what it can find on the internet rather than relying solely on its training data, the likelihood of hallucinations is meaningfully reduced. It's the difference between a medical student answering from memory and one who has access to a textbook during the exam.

Second, because the model is pulling from multiple sources, it can cross-check facts across those sources. This may further reduce errors. If three independent sources agree on a fact and one disagrees, the model can flag the discrepancy or hedge its answer accordingly. This built-in verification doesn't make the output infallible—after all, not everything you read on the internet is true—but it adds a layer of reliability that the default chat functionality lacks.

One way to use this feature is to power a literature search. Rather than manually searching PubMed, reading abstracts, taking notes, and then organizing those notes, you can give the AI model a research question and let it do the legwork. It will formulate the search queries, read the results, follow links, and compile a comprehensive summary—all with citations that you can verify.

For example, you might prompt:

> Search for the latest evidence on late effects of cranial radiation in pediatric ALL survivors. Focus on neurocognitive outcomes and any emerging screening recommendations. Provide citations for every claim.

The model will spend several minutes autonomously searching the web and reading the pages it finds, then present you with a structured summary grounded in what it found. This is not a replacement for a systematic review, but it can be used as a starting point to get up to speed on a particular topic and identify key references. A key strength of deep research over the basic chat functionality is that every claim is anchored to a specific source you can click through to—and you should. Carefully review each cited source to confirm it actually says what the summary claims it says before you rely on it.

The capabilities of deep research come with two important trade-offs you should be aware of.

The first is **time**. While a standard chat query returns a response in seconds, deep research and extended thinking queries can take five to fifteen minutes to process—sometimes longer for particularly complex questions. The model is doing real work: formulating search queries, reading pages, "reasoning" through what it found, and synthesizing the results. These are the kinds of tasks where you fire off the prompt and take a break to make a cup of coffee while the model works.

The second trade-off is **cost**. These queries consume significantly more tokens than standard interactions. The model is using tokens for its internal reasoning steps, for processing every webpage it reads, and for generating the final structured output. If you're on a metered subscription, these queries will eat through your usage allowance much faster, and if you're paying using an API (e.g., through OpenRouter) you'll pay more for these. This doesn't mean you shouldn't use them, as the value they provide often far exceeds the cost. You should be strategic about when to deploy them and ensure that your prompt is specific about what you want (and don't want). If you aren't careful, you can waste a bunch of tokens on a research project that goes in the opposite direction than the one you wanted. Save deep research for the complex questions that genuinely benefit from it, and use standard chat for the simple ones.

Similarly, most consumer AI platforms now include real-time web search as a standard feature. This use-case is the core feature of Perplexity, the LLM-powered search tool. When you ask a question, the model can search the web on the fly and ground its answer in what it finds. This addresses a key limitation: the model's training data has a cutoff date, but web search allows it to access information published after that cutoff. The key distinction between "deep research" and incorporation of web search is the depth of the search—the number of pages retrieved and reviewed in the latter use case is much smaller than in the former.

## Key Takeaways: Advanced Workflows

- Working with Files and “Lightweight RAG”: Upload files to create custom RAG systems that ground AI responses in your own documents and data.
- Personal Prompt Library: Build a prompt library—your "dot phrases" for the LLM—so you never have to retype your best prompts.
- AI "Memory": The system takes notes about you as you chat with it, and it can personalize responses.
- Connectors and Agents: Connect AI tools with other apps you already use. Be cautious: granting AI access permissions to other apps introduces data leakage risks.
- “Vibe Coding”: Anyone can write and edit computer code using natural language prompts.
- Deep research and Web-Grounded Search: The model searches the web and synthesizes results.

# Part IV: Safety, Security, and Accountability

# Chapter 12: Practical Security—Shadow IT and Accidental Oversharing

When we think about cybersecurity in healthcare, we might picture malicious hackers trying to lock down a hospital's electronic health record and demanding ransom in Bitcoin. But with AI, one of the most overlooked security threats might not be a hacker in a dark room. It could be a well-meaning, exhausted clinician at 5:00 PM trying to finish their notes so they can go home to their family.

**Shadow IT** refers to the hardware or software that employees use without the knowledge or approval of the organization's IT department. Generative AI has caused shadow IT to explode, and shadow IT can be problematic when it risks exposure of protected health information and sensitive business data.

It's tempting to find a cool new AI app on your phone, pay $20 with your personal credit card, and start using it to dictate your clinical notes or summarize a 300-page PDF file with outside hospital records. But when you do this, you are likely bypassing important privacy and security safeguards your hospital has invested in, and you may be violating the law.

As we've discussed before, it is crucial to be careful when entering PHI or sensitive business data into an LLM. You should understand the agreements that your employer has with a given LLM vendor before using it, and ensure a BAA is in place before entering PHI into an LLM. On the flip side, you may also wish to understand the extent to which your LLM chats are monitored and logged by your employer. Chances are, if your employer is providing an AI tool for your use, they can audit what has gone into that tool and what has come out. Don't put anything into that tool that you wouldn't want your employer seeing.

## Integrated AI Tools: What Could Possibly Go Wrong?

I'm going to review two key risks associated with integrated AI tools.

### 1. The Trojan Horse: Browser Extensions

There are countless "AI Assistant" extensions that you can install in your browser that promise to transform your life. They promise to live in your browser and summarize long articles, draft emails, and define complex terms for you, all with a single click (or maybe even automatically). Many LLM vendors (including OpenAI and Perplexity) have developed their own browsers that have this capability built in.

They sound incredibly helpful. But many of these free extensions and browsers have a dark side: they work by literally "reading" the webpages you browse, and they may track your browsing history.

Imagine you install one of these extensions on your work laptop to help you summarize websites. Later that afternoon, you log into your hospital email account via the web browser to review an email about a patient. That free, consumer-grade AI extension—built by an unknown developer, with no BAA in place—may have quietly read and processed that patient's PHI.

**The guardrail:** Never install unvetted third-party AI browser extensions on a computer you use for clinical care.

### 2. Connector Leakage

In the last chapter, we talked about how powerful it can be to connect an AI model to your email inbox or your calendar so it can act as your personal assistant.

The security risk here is called **data leakage**. If you give an AI model permission to read your email to summarize your inbox every morning, you have given it access to *all* of your emails.

What happens if you ask a connected AI model to summarize a research paper, but it gets confused and instead summarizes a highly confidential peer review email you received? What if it reads an email regarding a faculty disciplinary issue and accidentally incorporates that sensitive information into a departmental memo it drafts for you?

**The guardrail:** Keep AI tools and your inbox strictly separated, unless you are using an enterprise-grade tool that your employer explicitly manages and secures. Do not give a consumer AI app the keys to your professional life. Always proofread AI outputs before sharing them.

## A Message to Leadership: Give Your People the Right Tools

Everything I've written in this chapter so far has been directed at the individual clinician: be careful, follow the rules, and don't use unapproved tools. That's sage advice, and I stand by it.

But I also want to take this opportunity to make a direct plea to those of you in leadership—chief medical officers, chief medical informatics officers, chief information officers, department chairs, and anyone else with the authority to shape your organization's AI strategy. If you're reading this and thinking "Good—I hope my staff pays attention to the advice in this book, obeys the rules, and stops using unapproved AI tools," I'd ask you to reframe the issue entirely.

Shadow IT is not primarily a compliance problem. **It's a signal**. When employees work *around* official systems to get their work done, the most important question isn't *why are they violating policy*, it's *what do the unapproved tools have that the ones we're providing don't, and why do employees feel so compelled to use those tools instead?* Just as modern patient safety has shifted from punitively blaming individuals to critically examining the systems and conditions that make errors inevitable, we should apply the same lens to AI adoption. When a physician is asking a consumer chatbot to summarize a PDF full of disorganized records at midnight on a busy call shift, that's not purely a disciplinary issue—it's also a manifestation of a gap between the tools you've provided and the work that actually needs to get done.

Your staff are already using these tools for work. They're using them on their personal phones and personal laptops, outside the walls of your secured environment, because they are drowning in administrative burden and these tools provide a lifeline. You can write all the policies you want prohibiting unapproved AI use, but if you don't provide an approved alternative that actually meets their needs, those policies are likely to be ignored. You will have a shadow IT problem, no matter how many strongly worded memos you send.

The solution is to make high-quality AI tools available to your staff through a secured, enterprise-grade environment. And here's the part that many health systems get wrong: don't just pick the most convenient option from the software company you already have a contract with. The tool you offer needs to actually be *good*. It needs to be one of the best tools available—not a watered-down, enterprise-only product that feels like a downgrade from what your staff can get for $20 a month on their own.

If the AI tool you provide to your employees is clunky, slow, limited in capability, or produces noticeably inferior output compared to what they can access on their personal devices, they will continue using the unapproved tools in secret. The shadow IT problem will perpetuate because you've given them a "solution" that doesn't actually solve their problem. The organizational tool needs to match or exceed what's available on the consumer market, or your staff will find a way around it.

When you get this right, the benefits are enormous. You bring AI use out of the shadows and into a managed, HIPAA-compliant environment. You reduce risk. You reduce the likelihood that PHI ends up in an unapproved system. And you empower your clinicians to do their best work with the best tools available—which, at the end of the day, is good for everyone. Wouldn't you rather your physicians use AI in a secured environment that you manage and monitor, rather than on a personal app that you don't even know exists?

In the opening chapter, I advised readers not to get locked into one specific vendor. The AI landscape moves fast enough that today's leading model may be largely irrelevant within a year. This advice holds true for hospital IT administrators: avoid long-term contracts with any single vendor, and where possible, maintain relationships with multiple providers. The goal is to keep switching costs low so that when the next leap happens, your organization can move to the next best thing with as little friction as possible.

## Key Takeaways

- One of the most overlooked AI security threats in healthcare isn't a malicious hacker—it's a well-meaning, exhausted clinician using an unapproved tool to get work done.
- Never install unvetted AI browser extensions on a device used for clinical care; they may silently read and process PHI.
- Don't link AI tools to your work inbox unless secured and approved by your employer.
- Shadow IT is a signal, not just a compliance problem. It's a signal of a mismatch between what the organization is offering and the work that needs to be done. Leaders must provide high-quality, approved AI tools that match or exceed what staff can access on their own.
- Avoid long-term single-vendor contracts. The AI landscape moves fast, and switching costs should be kept low.

# Chapter 13: How AI Can Hurt Patients (and You)

We've spent several chapters talking about how incredibly capable AI is. It's fast, it's articulate, and it can synthesize vast amounts of data in seconds.

Now, we need to have a serious conversation about what happens when it fails in patient care applications.

In medicine, when a tool fails, it doesn't just result in a bad user experience. It can result in patient harm. Before you ever use an AI model to assist with a clinical task, you must keenly understand the specific ways these models can break down.

## 1. Bias and Transfer Failure

AI models are trained on historical data. Therefore, AI models inherit historical patterns and biases that are encoded in that historical data. If an LLM is trained predominantly on clinical notes written at an urban, academic medical center in Boston that cares primarily for adults, the patterns it learns from those notes might not apply as well to analysis of notes from a community-based practice in North Dakota that cares for a rural, pediatric population.

In machine learning, this is known as **transfer failure**. The algorithm looks like a genius in the environment where it was trained, but when you transfer it to a new environment with a different patient demographic, its accuracy plummets.

## 2. Automation Bias

Humans often follow the easiest path—the path of least resistance. I don't mean that as an insult; it's a well-established cognitive tendency. Work smarter—not harder—right?

When you use a tool that is accurate 99% of the time, your brain gradually stops double-checking the output. You learn to trust the machine. This is called **automation bias**.

Think about the drug-drug interaction alerts that pop up in your electronic medical record software. Have you ever instinctively clicked "dismiss" on an alert and then recognized that you didn't even read it? We develop this behavior because the false-positive rate for these notifications is so high that we develop alert fatigue, and we start ignoring the alerts. With AI, the output is usually so beautifully written, so confidently stated, and so highly structured that we might assume it *must* be correct, and we may not second-guess it. Then, when the rare hallucination inevitably happens, we miss it because we've outsourced our critical thinking to the computer and come to trust the model more than we should.

## 3. Administrative Harm and the "Note Bloat" Epidemic

Not all AI harm is directly clinical; some of it is administrative.

One of the most popular uses of AI in healthcare right now is ambient scribing—using AI to listen to a patient visit and automatically generate the clinical note. This is a fantastic technology that I use every day in the clinic.

But there is a dark side. Because AI can generate text instantly, it sometimes generates *too much* text and is too verbose. We are already suffering from **note bloat** thanks to note templates that pull in a variety of data from the medical record to make our notes look longer (and more detailed) than they actually need to be. If every doctor uses AI to generate three-page, highly detailed, beautifully formatted progress notes, it becomes impossible for the next doctor to find the actual clinical nugget buried inside all that synthetic text. Sometimes less is more.

With AI-driven note generation, we risk polluting the medical record with AI-generated filler. When the signal-to-noise ratio drops, important clinical details may get missed.

## The Guardrail

In modern medicine, the wealth of knowledge about human disease is exponentially greater than it ever used to be. It used to be that you went to the library stacks and used the Dewey Decimal System to find a book, found journal articles in bound issues on the periodicals shelf, and so much of the art of medicine was passed down orally from attending to trainee. Today, we face the challenge of an explosion of data, where the corpus of medical information could not physically fit in a local library, and it is impossible to memorize it all. While it's difficult for us to sift through all of that data, the explosion of data is overall a *good* thing for our patients—we understand their diseases and how to optimally treat them better than we ever have.

AI is a tool that will help us navigate that explosion. But it is just that: a navigation tool.

Think of it like the GPS in your car. It is incredibly useful for finding the fastest route to your destination. But if the GPS confidently tells you to turn right, and you can clearly see that turning right will drive your car directly into a lake (as happened on a memorable episode of *The Office*), you should not turn right.

Use AI for information retrieval, synthesis, and administrative leverage, but never, *ever* let it replace your final clinical judgment. You are the physician. You are the pilot, and AI is just the copilot. It doesn't have a medical license, it's not accountable to your patients, and it isn't exposed to legal liability the way you are when things go wrong.

## Key Takeaways

- AI models inherit biases from their training data. A model trained on one patient population may perform poorly when applied to a different demographic (transfer failure).
- Beware of automation bias: when a tool is accurate 99% of the time, your brain gradually stops double-checking—and that's when rare errors get through the holes in the proverbial Swiss cheese.
- AI-generated note bloat can bury clinically relevant details in verbose, synthetic text, making it harder for the next clinician to find what matters.
- Never let AI replace your final clinical judgment. You are the physician. You are the pilot. AI is just the copilot.

# Chapter 14: The Anatomy of a Perfect Lie (Hallucinated Citations)

I want to revisit the concept of hallucinations one more time, because this is where some of the smartest and most experienced physicians can get fooled.

If you ask an AI model, "What is the capital of France?" and it says "London," you instantly know it's wrong. The hallucination is obvious. But AI models are incredibly sophisticated pattern matchers. When they hallucinate, they often don't produce obvious nonsense. They produce highly plausible-sounding fiction, stated very confidently.

Let me give you a real-world example.

In my earliest days using an LLM, I asked ChatGPT to look up literature references. There was a fact I knew to be true, and I just needed help finding a verifiable source to cite. I used ChatGPT as a souped-up version of PubMed to help me with this task. For the specific concept I was seeking a reference to support, ChatGPT replied with a citation and a summary of the article. The last name and first initial of the author matched a world expert in the specific discipline, the title plausibly described a study that would be expected to include this fact, and the journal listed was a flagship journal of our discipline. It all seemed to check out. The problem was that if you looked up that article on the journal's website, it doesn't exist.

In essence, the model *knew* that an article that contains what I was looking for would likely have this style of title, be written by someone like the expert it cited, and be published in the flagship journal. But if you go to PubMed and search for the citation, the article does not exist. The model generated a reference that *looked* right for what I was asking for, but it was not based in truth and fact.

This is the autocomplete engine from Chapter 4 in action. The model wasn't searching a database of real articles. It was predicting, token by token, what a plausible citation *would look like* given the patterns it learned during training. The author name, the journal, the title—each was a statistically likely next token in the sequence. The result looked perfect, precisely because the model is excellent at matching patterns. It just wasn't matching reality.

Today's LLMs are addressing this issue by grounding their results in search and using RAG, as we discussed in Chapters 6 and 11, yet even use of these systems requires manual verification.

## Misinformation and Bias: Why Hallucinations Are Not the Only Problem

The accuracy of an LLM output is directly related to the accuracy of both the training data and, when RAG or web search is used, the reference data the model retrieves at query time. Even current models that ground their results in search are susceptible to this flaw. Models rely on data from the internet, which can hardly be considered the *de facto* source of truth. Some sources have trusted provenance (e.g., academic medical journals), but others may be questionable (e.g., "predatory" medical journals, online forums, and social media). These sources can perpetuate biases that they contain and can include misinformation that gets embedded into the LLM. This is one reason why a curated

RAG pipeline—that references only trusted sources—is among the most promising ways to use AI in healthcare and other knowledge fields that require high reliability based on a defined source of truth.

## The Standard Workflow for Verification

**The guardrail:** You must adopt a zero-tolerance policy for hallucinated citations. If you are using AI to help with literature reviews, grant writing, or manuscript drafting, you must use this standard workflow:

1. **Demand structure:** In your prompt, tell the AI model, *"For every claim you make, provide a citation. Include the PMID (PubMed Unique Identifier) or a DOI (Digital Object Identifier)."*
2. **Verify existence:** Do not just read the title and nod. Copy the PMID or DOI and paste it into PubMed. Prove the paper actually exists.
3. **Read the primary source:** Finally, just because the paper exists doesn't mean the AI model summarized it correctly. The model might cite a real paper that concluded a drug was *ineffective*, but hallucinate a summary saying the drug was *effective*. Read the paper and see what it says.

If you do not have the time to verify a citation against the primary source, you should not be using AI for that task. Always aggressively verify.

## Key Takeaways

- Hallucinated citations are especially dangerous because they look plausible: a real expert's name, a believable title, and a flagship journal.
- Even when models ground results in web search, deep research or RAG, manual verification of every citation is required.
- Adopt a zero-tolerance workflow: demand structured citations with PMIDs or DOIs, verify that each paper exists, and read the primary source to confirm accuracy before citing the source.
- Misinformation from low-quality sources on the internet can be embedded in model outputs even when RAG is used, leading to inaccurate outputs.

# Chapter 15: The Rules of Disclosure

This brings us to a very practical question: if you use AI to help you do your work, do you need to tell people? If so, what level of detail about your use is appropriate?

The answer depends on how you are using AI.

**Shades of gray:** I would imagine that if you polled 100 people with the following two questions, they would give pretty uniform answers. (1) If you use AI to spellcheck an email, do you need to disclose it? (2) If you ask AI to write a book for you, it writes the entire book on its own, and you publish it as the author without making any substantive edits or revisions, should you disclose it? Most would suggest that AI spellcheck does not need to be disclosed, as these tools have been in standard use for decades to the extent that their use is *expected* by default. But to pass off wholly AI-generated content as one's own work goes too far. The reality is that most uses of AI—in particular, the most creative, effective, and collaborative uses—are going to fall somewhere between these extremes. Standards for disclosing the role of AI have been proposed and are surely going to develop and mature over time. My opinion after reading a thoughtful article by David Resnik and Mohammad Hosseini[1] is that the extent to which AI use should be disclosed is directly proportional to (1) the extent

---

[1]Resnik DB, Hosseini M. Disclosing artificial intelligence use in scientific research and publication: When should disclosure be mandatory, optional, or unnecessary? Accountability in Research. 2026;33(2):2481949. doi:10.1080/08989621.2025.2481949

of AI use and (2) the impact of AI use on the substance of the output.

There is another dimension to disclosure that goes beyond professional norms: intellectual honesty. Using AI is not inherently problematic—as I argue throughout this book, it can meaningfully improve the quality of your work. But when you present AI-generated ideas, analysis, or reasoning as if they originated entirely from your own thinking, you are misrepresenting the origin of those ideas. You could consider this to be similar to plagiarism. The two primary issues with plagiarism are that (1) the original author doesn't receive credit, and (2) the credit is falsely attributed to the listed author. With AI, it's primarily this second issue that's at hand. The reader assumes they are seeing the product of your expertise and reasoning, when in reality, parts of that product were generated or substantially shaped by a machine. The principle to follow here is the same one we teach about citing sources: make it clear where the ideas came from and how they were developed.

What this really is about is trust and accountability. A patient would likely be upset if a response to a message to their doctor was completely AI-generated and a human in the clinic didn't even bother to review it. Yet, they likely would *not* be upset if their physician used an AI tool to flag medical jargon in their draft message and then suggested to the physician ways they could improve readability and understandability. It's where cases fall between the extremes that the lines become blurry. When AI is used, it is helpful for the reader to understand *what the AI tool did* versus *what the human author did*. Did the AI tool write a first draft of a manuscript from scratch? Did it proofread and critique your initial human-written draft?

I think of AI like a good editor. If you've ever worked with an editor on a publication, you know the relationship: the editor helps shape the structure, proposes cuts and additions, catches errors, tightens the prose, and sometimes pushes you to rethink your argument entirely. A great editor makes the work dramatically better. But the byline belongs to the author, because the final work product belongs to the author, and the author is accountable for the finished product. Nobody assumes an author works without editorial input, and nobody thinks less of the work because an editor improved it. What matters is that the person whose name is on it did the substantive intellectual work and took ownership of the result.

AI works the same way. It can help you think through ideas, draft your work, organize your ideas, and propose approaches you might not have considered. But ultimately, what you present to the world—the note you sign, the grant you submit, and the recommendation you make to a family—is your decision. You are accountable for it.

Many AI use disclosure guidelines also suggest that the specific model or models used be disclosed. While I can understand the rationale underlying this practice, I would also argue that the specific model or models used is far less important than disclosure of AI use at all. This is because these models do not provide the same exact outputs for a given set of inputs. If you are describing a science experiment, it is recommended to disclose which manufacturer provided the reagents so that another scientist could replicate the experiment in the exact same way you did it, but AI models don't work this way. You wouldn't expect someone to try rewriting your research manuscript from scratch using an AI model to see if they ended up with the same result. What is most crucial is that a human is accountable for the output and that AI use is honestly disclosed.

**In academic writing:** The rules here have crystallized rapidly. Almost all major medical journals now have explicit AI disclosure policies. The consensus is that an AI model *cannot* be listed as a co-author because it cannot take legal or ethical responsibility for the work. If you use AI to help draft a manuscript, translate text, or analyze data, you are expected to explicitly disclose use of AI.

**In peer review:** The use of AI in peer review raises its own set of concerns. A peer reviewer who pastes a manuscript into an AI tool to generate their review is potentially exposing unpublished, confidential research to a third-party vendor—a serious breach of the trust that underpins the peer review process. Beyond confidentiality, there is another substantive concern: peer review is valued precisely because it reflects the informed judgment of a domain expert. If a reviewer outsources that judgment to a model that lacks true domain expertise and may hallucinate critiques or miss field-specific nuances, the quality and integrity of the review process is compromised. If you use AI to assist with peer review—for example, to help organize your thoughts or check whether you've addressed all sections of a manuscript—do so transparently, follow the journal's AI use policy, and ensure that the final review reflects your own expert assessment. Never upload confidential manuscripts to AI tools without explicit permission from the journal and authors. If you have permission to upload the manuscript to an LLM, ensure training using user data is turned off.

**Have no shame:** I want to be very direct here about something. When AI disclosure requirements first appeared, the subtext was clear: if you used AI, you should be a little embarrassed about it. The framing suggested that AI-assisted work was lesser work—that admitting you used these tools was akin to admitting you couldn't do it on your own. It was treated less like a standard methodological disclosure and more like a confession. As I've very honestly and openly disclosed with this book (starting with the prologue), I used AI to help organize my thoughts, perform research, draft the first version, and copyedit the final version—with countless hours of manual revision over several weeks between each AI-assisted step. This was a collaborative and iterative process. I prompted AI to help me think about how certain concepts are explained or how the book is structured, reviewed the options and suggestions it made, and decided on the final course of action. I have no shame in admitting this, and I strongly believe that AI has *improved* the quality of the work, rather than *cheapened* it. AI resulted in a better product *for you*, the reader. By now, you're getting close to the end of the book. Based on what you've read so far, do you think AI helped me put out a better product, or an inferior one?

**In clinical documentation:** Hospitals generally reject statements at the end of clinical notes that attempt to escape accountability for transcription errors when the author has used speech-to-text tools to dictate notes. Ultimately, the physician is responsible and accountable for the content of the signed note, regardless of how it was generated. These disclaimers provide little practical function other than to alert readers that the physician may be sloppy in their documentation, as they are relying on a disclaimer to make up for their failure to proofread. When ambient scribe technology is used, it is important to obtain consent from the parties who were recorded and to indicate that consent was obtained. Regardless of what the ambient scribe software generates, the physician alone is responsible and accountable for the content of the signed note. When I use an ambient scribe, I indicate that consent was obtained and that the note was drafted with the assistance of AI not to disclaim any liability for errors, but to provide transparency.

**A critical caveat:** The conventions, standards, and professional expectations around AI disclosure are rapidly evolving. Always follow your institution's policies, procedures and all applicable laws and regulations. Regardless of how standards about AI use evolve, one principle will remain constant: *you* are ultimately responsible and accountable for any work product that bears your name.

## Key Takeaways

- The extent of AI disclosure depends on the extent and impact of AI use on the substance of the output.
- Think of AI like a good editor: it helps to shape, suggest, and refine, but the byline—and the accountability—belongs to you.
- In academic writing, AI cannot be listed as a co-author. Disclose its use explicitly in accordance with journal policies.
- Take caution when using AI to assist with manuscript peer review. Always follow journal policies, disclose AI use, and do not upload confidential peer review manuscripts to an LLM without the permission of the author and journal.
- Have no shame in disclosing AI use. The question is not whether you used AI, but whether you took ownership, applied judgment, and are ultimately accountable for the result.
- In clinical documentation, the physician is responsible for the signed note, regardless of how it was generated. Disclosure should provide transparency and not seek to act as a disclaimer of liability for errors.

# Part V: The Playbook

# Chapter 16: Healthcare Use Cases Organized by Risk

We have covered the mechanics, the prompt engineering, the risks, the safety guardrails and the rules of disclosure. Now, it's time to put it all together.

When colleagues ask me, "How should I actually use this on Monday morning?" I always categorize the use cases by risk. If you are new to employing AI in your work, you must start at the bottom of the ladder and only climb to the top of the risk ladder when you have mastered the guardrails.

## Tier 1: Low Risk, High Value—Start Here

These are tasks where a hallucination is highly unlikely to harm a patient, but the time saved for the clinician is immense.

- **Administrative Correspondence:** Drafting letters of medical necessity or writing prior authorization denial appeal letters. Don't feel guilty—insurance companies are increasingly using AI to generate their own denial letters.
- **Scheduling and Logic:** *"Here are the vacation requests for the six fellows in my division, and here are the rules for who can be off at the same time. Draft a workable call schedule with these existing vacation requests. Identify any conflicts."*
- **Text-to-Speech Audio Consumption:** Using text-to-speech tools to listen to articles and documents during your daily commute.

## Tier 2: Medium Risk—Requires Aggressive Verification

In this tier, you are asking the AI model to process clinical or scientific data. The negative consequences of hallucinations increase, so your verification must be airtight.

- **Literature Reviews:** Ask the AI model to summarize the state of the art for a specific disease—perhaps a rare disease or a rare disease presentation for which no comprehensive, well-organized review exists. You must use the verification workflow we discussed in Chapter 14 to check every single citation.
- **Chart Abstraction:** Let's say you receive an 800-page PDF of disorganized outside hospital records for a new consult. We've all been on the receiving end of these enormous packets with every hemoglobin level printed on a new page and the same progress note included three times. Rather than manually sifting through these, you could upload the PDF into an enterprise, BAA-covered AI tool and ask: *"Create a timeline of every chemotherapy agent this patient received, and list their highest and lowest creatinine levels."* This can be helpful as you prepare for the visit, but you should not copy and paste the AI model's output directly into your own note without manually checking the source pages and verifying important details with the patient. A similar approach could potentially be used for medical record abstraction in chart review research studies, significantly decreasing manual chart abstraction burden.

## Tier 3: High Risk—Use as a Sparring Partner

This is the top of the ladder: diagnostic reasoning and medical decision-making.

You should never ask an AI system, *"What is wrong with this patient?"* and just accept its answer. Instead, leverage AI to combat your own cognitive biases. Use it as a sparring partner. Use it to poke holes in your differential diagnosis and medical reasoning. Make sure you are using an employer-approved, BAA-covered tool and following all applicable privacy laws and the policies and procedures of your organization before entering any patient-specific information into an LLM.

If you have a complex patient who isn't responding to standard therapy, you can type a de-identified presentation into such a tool and ask: *"My leading diagnosis is X. What am I missing? Give me three diagnoses that fit this clinical picture but are unrelated to X. Point out the flaws in my current reasoning."*

Used this way, the AI model doesn't make the diagnosis for you. It forces you to broaden your differential. It makes you think more critically. It acts as a tireless, highly read colleague who is not afraid to disagree with you.

## Key Takeaways

- Start at the bottom of the risk ladder: administrative correspondence, scheduling logic, and audio consumption of articles are low-risk, high-value use cases.
- Medium-risk uses—like literature reviews and chart abstraction—require aggressive verification of every claim and citation.
- At the top of the ladder, use AI as a sparring partner for diagnostic reasoning: challenge your own differential, but don't accept the model's answer uncritically.
- Always follow your institution's policies, procedures and applicable laws when entering patient-specific information into any AI tool.

# Chapter 17: Rolling Out AI in Health Systems

If you are a clinical leader, a medical director, or just someone who wants to champion AI in your department, using AI on your personal laptop isn't enough. You have to figure out how to deploy it across an entire organization and integrate employer-approved tools.

As a clinical informatician, I can tell you that rolling out AI is not primarily an IT challenge—it's mostly an administrative and change-management challenge. The tools already exist; the challenge is getting them into the hands of the right people and helping them use those tools on the right tasks in sensible, safe, and effective ways. That is, in large part, why I wrote this book—to help clinicians integrate these tools into their workflows thoughtfully. Here is how health systems can approach it from the organizational side, while ensuring all appropriate security and privacy safeguards are in place.

## 1. The Right Pilots

Do not start your hospital's AI journey by trying to diagnose ultra-rare diseases or find a universal cure for cancer. Don't try to boil the ocean.

Instead, start with a pilot that tackles the most universally despised administrative burden you can find. Ambient scribing—where AI listens to the visit and drafts the note—is the perfect Trojan horse to get clinicians using AI. Its adoption has expanded dramatically over the past couple of years. When doctors are provided tools that improve their workflows, they will become champions and believers in the technology.

And as I discussed in Chapter 12, choose the *best* tools for these pilots, not just the most convenient ones. If you pilot ambient scribing with a mediocre tool and your clinicians have a bad first experience, you've just created a building full of AI skeptics and your next AI rollout will be met with resistance. First impressions matter. Invest in the right tools upfront, and your early adopters will become your most effective evangelists.

## 2. Beware of Model Drift

When you buy a new ultrasound machine, the pictures you get on day 1,000 look similar to the pictures you got on day 1. AI models do not do this. They experience **model drift**. The companies that build these models are constantly tweaking the underlying algorithms with the goal of improving them. A prompt that extracted data perfectly in January might suddenly start hallucinating in July because the vendor updated the model.

Separately, even when the model itself hasn't changed, its accuracy can shift as the real-world patient data it sees changes over time (e.g., due to population changes). This change in model performance is called **data drift**.

You cannot deploy an AI tool and forget about it. You can't "set it and forget it." You must establish continuous monitoring of system performance to ensure the models continue to function as well—if not better—on day 1,000 as compared to on day 1.

## 3. Human-in-the-Loop Governance

Finally, your hospital must establish AI governance policies along with a governing committee. This cannot just be the Chief Information Officer, Chief Medical Informatics Officer, and a few software developers. It should include frontline attending physicians, nurses, pharmacists, legal counsel, and risk-management and compliance officers.

Every AI workflow deployed in your system should be designed with a "human in the loop" before action is taken. The software should make it easy to generate a draft, but it should introduce intentional friction before that draft becomes permanent. The physician must always be the final gatekeeper, forced to review and sign their name.

If we design our systems so that the AI does the heavy lifting, but the clinician provides the final layer of judgment, we can more safely navigate this transition and fundamentally improve the way we practice medicine.

## Key Takeaways

- Start AI pilots with universally despised administrative burdens (like documentation), not moonshot clinical applications. First impressions matter.
- Choose the *best* tools for pilots, not just the most convenient. A bad first experience creates a building full of AI skeptics.
- AI models experience drift. Model drift occurs when the vendor updates the underlying model. Data drift occurs when the population the model is being applied to changes over time. Establish continuous monitoring plans.
- AI governance should include frontline clinicians, nurses, pharmacists, legal counsel, and compliance officers—not just IT leadership.
- Design every AI workflow with a human in the loop and intentional friction before any AI-generated output becomes permanent.

# Part VI: The Future and Staying Current

# Chapter 18: What's Next—Proteins, Drugs, and Synthetic Documentation

If you read the tech blogs, you might be hearing hype that a new AI model is going to arrive next week, instantly cure all known diseases, and render doctors entirely obsolete.

As a clinician and an informatician, I don't buy the hype. However, I am incredibly optimistic about where the trajectory is pointing. The chatbots you use today are only one application of the underlying architecture; the same family of models is starting to be applied more broadly.

Here are two areas where I think AI will be transformative for our field over the next five years—and one looming risk we need to prepare for.

## 1. Biology as a Language

Think back to our discussion on how LLMs work. They ingest massive sequences of words, map the statistical relationships between them, and learn to predict what comes next.

Now, ask yourself: what else in biology is just a massive sequence of letters in recurring patterns?

DNA. RNA. Amino acids.

Companies like EvolutionaryScale have realized that you can treat biology like a language. Over 20 years ago, the Human Genome Project aimed to map the human genome. The wealth of information we have collected on sequence variants and protein function has become a Rosetta Stone for decoding the language of nature.

Just like ChatGPT can write a completely novel poem that has never existed before, these biological AI models can design completely novel proteins that do not exist in nature. EvolutionaryScale's ESM3 model developed a novel green fluorescent protein that shares relatively little in common with previously discovered green fluorescent proteins yet functions by emitting green fluorescence like ones that exist in nature. According to the research team, the model took a leap that the authors estimate would have taken evolution on the order of 500 million years to achieve—an extraordinary claim that underscores the potential, even if the precise timeline involves significant assumptions. The implications of this are huge. We are moving toward an era where we could envision designing a novel and highly specific biological molecule to bind to a mutated protein in a cancer cell. In the future, we may be able to generate completely custom drugs in a fraction of the time the drug development process currently takes.

## 2. Healthcare-Specific Foundation Models

Right now, we are mostly taking models trained on the public internet and applying them to medical tasks.

The truth is that the language of the internet is very different from that of clinical notes, radiology reports, and pathology reports. In the future, we will hopefully welcome models trained on a diverse set of native healthcare data spanning clinical notes, clinical and radiology images, histology slides, genomic and other -omic sequences, structured laboratory and vital sign data, and social determinants of health. Models trained on real healthcare data will be able to understand and encode patient trajectories in ways that allow us to predict patient outcomes using real-world healthcare data better than we can with off-the-shelf general-purpose language models.

The primary hurdle will not be the technology; it's going to be the privacy, governance, and de-identification of that massive amount of data.

## 3. The Risk: The Synthetic Feedback Loop

I want to end this chapter with a warning about a looming problem: the **synthetic feedback loop**.

Remember how we talked about ambient scribes and note bloat? AI is incredibly good at generating human-like output because it was trained on human output. But what happens over the next decade, when the majority of notes in the electronic health record are generated by AI? How good will AI trained on that AI-generated content be?

When the *next* generation of AI is trained on our medical records, it won't be learning from physician-generated notes that reflect complex clinical reasoning. It will be learning from the outputs of previous AI models—content increasingly distant from the bedside reasoning of an actual clinician, and increasingly the product of statistical patterns recombining prior model output. In computer science, this is called **model collapse**. It's like making a photocopy of a photocopy of a photocopy. Each generation, the sharp edges of clinical intuition get a little blurrier—until eventually the end product is illegible.

This is why provenance—knowing what is human-written and what is AI-generated—will become an important issue in clinical documentation over the next decade.

## Key Takeaways

- AI is being applied to biological sequences (DNA, RNA, amino acids) the same way LLMs process language, enabling the design of novel proteins and potentially custom drugs.
- Healthcare-specific foundation models trained on native clinical data—rather than the public internet—are likely to dramatically improve AI's ability to understand clinical language and patient trajectories.
- The synthetic feedback loop is a looming risk: as AI-generated notes fill medical records, future models trained on that synthetic content may lose the clinical nuance present in human-authored documentation. Provenance—knowing what is human-written and what is AI-generated—will become an important issue in clinical documentation.

# Chapter 19: Will AI Erode Critical Thinking? Only If You Let It.

A complaint I frequently hear is this: *"If we give these tools to our trainees, they will forget how to think critically."*

It's a valid fear. How will an intern ever build the cognitive muscle memory required to be an attending if they can click a button and have AI instantly summarize a 200-page chart, suggest a differential diagnosis, pre-order the initial laboratory workup, and draft the progress note?

My answer is that AI will only erode critical thinking if we misuse it. It will erode critical thinking if we use it to *replace* our critical thinking instead of using it to *augment* it.

Consider the calculator. When it was first introduced, you could imagine math teachers worried that students would no longer become proficient in arithmetic. And they were partially right—I can't tell you when I last performed multiplication or long division by hand; I reflexively reach for a calculator to do even simple math I could do in my head because using one has become a habit. But why *wouldn't* I use a calculator if it can offload the task from my brain and allow me to perform calculations more quickly and accurately than by hand? My mental arithmetic atrophied—and that's a real cost—but the cognitive bandwidth I freed up got reinvested in higher-level work I couldn't have done otherwise. That trade-off is the one we're negotiating with AI.

Calculators didn't destroy mathematics. Instead, they allowed us to move past tedious arithmetic and tackle higher-level calculus, physics, and engineering. Rather than spending a minute performing long division, we got the answer in a millisecond on a calculator and spent the time saved on other high-level tasks.

Similarly, the transition from paper charts to the electronic health record, and the rise of internet resources, have changed how we practice. We no longer memorize the exact dosing of every single antibiotic. We offloaded that storage to a database and look it up when we need it.

Generative AI is the next evolution of this cognitive offloading. It will enable us to leverage massive datasets to improve the lives of our patients. However, to do so in a way that is safe and effective, we must understand the underpinnings of the tools that are propping us up. We must understand what lies behind the curtain so that we can interpret its output. Just like with lab values, we need to know the reasons why a lab result we weren't expecting could be spurious. It's not that we can't use these tools—we just have to develop the skill of critically appraising them and assessing their results.

We don't lament the days before we had powerful tools to help us do this work; we have those tools now, and we should use them. We don't need to spend two hours reading through an unorganized stack of outside faxes just to find the date of a patient's last bone marrow biopsy. An AI system can do that and show you where it found the answer. Our critical thinking and cognitive effort shifts from *information gathering* to *information synthesis and judgment*. It enables us to spend our focus and attention on higher-level tasks.

## Stay Focused When You Use These Tools

There's an irony buried in the way these tools work that I think is worth pausing on, because it has changed how I approach AI in my own use.

In the world of computer hardware, CPUs—central processing units—have traditionally been the brains of computers. They are incredibly good at performing complex tasks, but they do them *sequentially*: one task at a time, completing each before starting the next. When a computer appears to "multitask," its CPU is actually bouncing rapidly between different tasks and doing each rapidly, one-at-a-time, giving the illusion of parallelism. The revolution that enabled large language models wasn't the CPU; it was the GPU—the graphics processing unit. GPUs were initially developed to display computer graphics. The difference between CPUs and GPUs is that GPUs can't handle tasks as complex as what a CPU can handle, but they excel at performing many relatively simple mathematical calculations *simultaneously*, in parallel. This parallel processing is what makes LLMs possible and why GPUs are the workhorses running them.

I think of our brains like CPUs. We're really not good at multitasking, even though we sometimes think we are. What we're actually doing is rapidly context-switching—bouncing between tasks—and each switch carries a cost in attention, accuracy, and depth of thought. When I use AI, I've noticed a temptation to treat it like an opportunity to multitask: fire off a prompt, then switch to my inbox while it processes, then jump back to read the response. Each time I switch, I lose a bit of the focused attention that would have helped me critically evaluate the AI's output.

The clinicians who want to get the most out of AI should resist this temptation. When you're working with an AI model, stay present in that conversation. Read its output carefully. Think about whether it's correct. Ask yourself whether it missed something. If you treat your interaction with AI as a focused, mindful dialogue—the way you would treat a conversation with a colleague whose opinion you're actively probing—you'll catch more errors, produce better work, and—I believe—actually strengthen your critical thinking rather than eroding it. If you instead treat AI as background noise while you bounce between mindless distractions, you will get exactly the shallow, uncritical outcome you fear, and your critical thinking will be eroded.

**The key insight is this: the risk to critical thinking doesn't come from the tool itself. It comes from how you use it.** If you use AI as an excuse to be less present, less focused, and less engaged, then yes, it will likely erode your thinking. But if you use it as an opportunity to focus your cognitive energy on higher-level reasoning—letting it handle the information gathering while you do the synthesis and judgment—my opinion is that it will make you sharper, not duller.

## Implications for Medical Education

This has direct implications for medical education. Training programs—residencies, fellowships, and medical schools—must incorporate AI literacy into their curricula. Programs that bury their heads in the proverbial sand and pretend AI doesn't exist are doing their trainees a disservice. Their graduates will enter the workforce alongside peers who understand how to use these tools safely and effectively, and they will be disadvantaged if they don’t know how to leverage them. Don't ban AI tools; instead, teach trainees how to effectively use them. The goal isn't to teach trainees to depend on AI; it's to teach them how to wield it as a tool while maintaining the foundational clinical reasoning skills that AI is designed to augment, not replace.

We've seen this pattern before with technology. Social media promised to connect us, but for many, it became a source of distraction and disconnection—mindless and endless scrolling at the dinner table instead of deeply personal conversation. AI could have the same effect if we let it become just another screen to stare at. But if used intentionally, AI is different: it's a tool that can give you time *back* rather than take it away. My hope is that AI helps you reclaim the mental effort you spend on tedious tasks so you can be more present in the moments that matter.

## Key Takeaways

- AI will erode critical thinking only if we use it to *replace* our thinking instead of *augmenting* it.
- When using AI, the cognitive effort shifts from gathering information to synthesizing it and critically thinking.
- Medical training programs must teach AI literacy. Banning these tools does trainees a disservice; teaching them to use AI effectively while maintaining foundational reasoning skills is essential.
- Stay focused and present when using AI. Treat it as a mindful dialogue, not background noise.
- The risk to critical thinking comes from *how you use the tool*, not from the tool itself.

# Chapter 20: A Closing Challenge

We have covered a lot of ground. We've talked about tokens, APIs, RAG, hallucinations, ambient scribing, and the future of drug discovery. I hope you've learned at least one or two things you didn't know before reading this book. I hope the hands-on experience—trying different models, adjusting the knobs, modifying prompts—has deepened your understanding of how these tools work.

Now that we're at the end, I'll let you in on something: I intentionally asked you to buy more OpenRouter credits than you'd need to complete the exercises in this book. That was by design. To effectively leverage the benefits AI promises, you have to build muscle memory. As I said in Chapter 1, **the only way to get better at using AI is to actually use it: early, often, and on a variety of tasks**. I wanted you to have credits left over so you'd have an excuse to keep experimenting. After all, *it sure would be a huge shame if you let those credits go to waste.* As of this writing, OpenRouter credits expire after a year, so keep tinkering with these LLMs. Compare different models, try the latest models as soon as they come out, and use AI to offload tedious tasks. Practice prompt engineering and try to push the boundaries to see exactly what high-performing AI can do for you.

I want to leave you with a 7-day challenge to help you use these credits. One week, one small task per day. You don't have to follow these instructions step by step. Instead, treat these as examples of ways you can try using AI tools. Try to use AI to do something new you've never done with it before each day, and start pushing the boundaries.

- **Day 1: The Polish.** Take a rough email or a messy set of ideas and ask an AI tool to organize it and correct the grammar while preserving your voice. Be as specific as you can in your prompt about what you want the output to look like and the tone and subtext you want to convey.
- **Day 2: The Prompt Library.** Identify one repetitive administrative task you detest. Write a structured prompt (Role, Task, Context, Constraints, and Format) to handle it, and save it in a document for future use. Use the prompt next time the task comes up. If there is something you don't like about the output, refine the prompt iteratively until you get it working exactly as you want.
- **Day 3: The Translation.** Take a complex medical concept—like a diagnosis, or how a drug works—and ask the AI model to explain it at a 6th-grade reading level for a patient. How does this explanation compare to the one you usually give in your office? Are there ways you could change the way you convey this information to patients?
- **Day 4: The Open Book Test.** Take a dense document, upload it to an AI model with a file-reading feature, and ask it three specific questions about the document. Compare the AI model's responses to your manual review.
- **Day 5: The Meeting or Visit Summary.** If your institution allows it, use an AI transcription tool or ambient scribe to capture a meeting or a patient visit and generate summary documentation.
- **Day 6: The Sparring Partner.** Bring a complex clinical case scenario to an employer-approved version of an advanced model that can safely handle PHI. Tell it your leading diagnosis, and ask it to argue against you.
- **Day 7: The Personal Policy—Making a Commitment.** Sit down and write your own rules of engagement. What will

you use AI for now and how will it improve your workflows over the next three months? What are your principles and guidelines for use? Now, choose a vendor and spend $20 on a one-month subscription. Immediately after subscribing, turn off auto-renew. Use it as you wish, and let me know at **kirk@aicurbsidebook.com** if you end up going back into settings to turn auto-renew back on. That button click tells you everything.

# Epilogue: The Final Word

Medicine is a fundamentally human endeavor. Patients don't just come to us for data processing. They come to us for empathy, judgment, and to serve as a trusted guide during some of the most uncertain moments of their lives.

Yuval Noah Harari, when referring to the application of AI, said, "Intelligence is the ability to solve problems. Wisdom is the ability to know which problems to solve." Harari is echoing an idea Aristotle worked out more than two thousand years ago. In *The Nicomachean Ethics*, Aristotle distinguished three kinds of knowledge. *Technē* was technical skill—the productive know-how to make something according to learned patterns. *Sophia* was theoretical wisdom, the deeper grasp of universal truths and the *why* behind them. And *phronēsis* was practical wisdom, the capacity to deliberate about what to do in a particular situation and in a particular moment. Aristotle considered *phronēsis* the master virtue, because without it, even vast knowledge could not be translated into good action. Critically, he argued that *phronēsis* cannot be acquired from study alone; it requires lived experience that only time can provide.

Aristotle's framework maps uncannily onto the AI era we are entering. Frontier AI models have something approaching *technē* on a scale Aristotle could never have imagined. They have developed extraordinary pattern-matching capabilities to create outputs at superhuman speed by drawing on vast amounts of training data. That capability is no longer scarce; anyone can access it. What these models do *not* have is the *understanding* behind *sophia* or the *judgment* behind *phronēsis*. They can produce outputs that imitate the products of both—a textbook-quality explanation, or a clinical recommendation that sounds like it came from a seasoned physician—but the imitation is statistical rather than substantive. The model has learned the pattern of what a confident answer *looks like* without any grasp of whether the answer is actually true, and without any capacity to weigh whether this answer is appropriate in *this* circumstance, in *this* moment.

You bring something fundamentally different to medicine. Medical school gave you something approaching *sophia*: a mental model of how the human body works. You aren't pattern matching when you reason through a case; you are drawing on a structured understanding of human anatomy, physiology and pharmacology that lets you predict what will happen and explain why. And your years on the wards and the sum of your human interactions over the course of your life have built in you something approaching *phronēsis*: the judgment to know what to do in a particular situation.

The intelligence—the *technē*—is available to anyone willing to pay for it. What distinguishes the clinician who thrives in this era is the *sophia* and *phronēsis* the machine cannot replicate. These tools are intelligent, but they are not wise. Anyone can use the intelligence; the wisest will apply it best.

What does that look like in practice? Three things we bring to patients are beyond the reach of any model:

**Trust.** The relationship between a clinician and a patient is built slowly through shared experiences that expose our vulnerabilities. AI systems may become familiar to us, and we may come to rely on them, but familiarity is not the same as trust. The bond a family develops with the physician guiding them through a cancer diagnosis is forged from something AI cannot replicate: the knowledge that another human being has chosen to show up, again and again, and that the outcome matters to them personally.

**Accountability.** If trust is about the relationship, accountability is about who owns the outcome. When I tell a family that their child has cancer and outline a prolonged treatment plan that involves toxic medications and no guarantee of cure, I am not just delivering information; I am taking responsibility for a course of action. That accountability is not incidental to what we do; it is central to it. An AI system can inform, recommend, and assist, but it cannot be held accountable.

**Humanness.** OK, this one is obvious—AI isn't human. Let me ask you this: which has a greater impact, a handwritten thank-you note or a brief email with the same words? The handwritten note is more impactful because the act of taking time to handwrite it gave it a human touch and showed that the writer cared. When I sit down with families to share difficult news, I've found I often don't say much. I share the news, and then I remain quiet while a wave of emotions comes over the family. In that moment, the role we play as physicians is not the words we convey; it's our physical presence. While I strongly believe that these tools will enable us to be better physicians, it is naïve to think that they will replace this human element of what we do. It is true that AI models have been found to generate responses that patients perceive as more empathic and easier to understand, but they are not genuine. They are not human.

AI is here, and it is powerful, but it is just a tool. It is not your replacement. *You* are the clinician. *You* are in the driver's seat. Use this technology to clear away the administrative friction, handle tedious tasks, and help you manage massive amounts of data your brain is incapable of processing on its own. Then, get back to doing the deeply human work that drew you to medicine.

None of us went into medicine for the administrative tasks; we did it because we're scientifically curious and because we value deeply human connections. I firmly believe that will never change.

Thank you for taking this journey with me. I hope you feel more prepared to put these tools to work in your daily life. Now, go get behind the wheel and drive.

# Continue the Conversation

If this book has been useful to you, the best way to pay it forward is to mention it to a colleague who might benefit from it and leave a review wherever you purchase books online. Word of mouth and honest reviews make an enormous difference for independent authors like me, and they're how books like this find the people who need them most.

I'd love to hear from you directly. I welcome your comments and suggestions at kirk@aicurbsidebook.com.

If you'd like to stay up to date on AI in healthcare, visit my website at thecurbside.ai.

Thank you for reading.

# Glossary

**Agentic**—Describes AI behavior in which the model acts as an agent performing tasks on your behalf—such as reading your calendar, drafting emails, or executing multistep workflows—rather than simply responding to a single chat prompt.

**API (Application Programming Interface)**—A standardized way for software systems to communicate with each other. APIs allow applications to send prompts to and receive responses from language models programmatically.

**Automation bias**—The tendency for humans to over-rely on automated systems, gradually stopping double-checking outputs because the system is usually correct—making it more likely that rare errors will be missed.

**Business Associate Agreement (BAA)**—A legal contract between a healthcare organization and a technology vendor guaranteeing the vendor will protect patient data in accordance with HIPAA. A BAA is required before sharing protected health information with an AI vendor.

**Context window**—The maximum number of tokens a model can hold in its working memory at any one time. Conversations that exceed this limit may lose earlier details through truncation or summarization.

**Data drift**—A gradual shift in the real-world inputs fed to an AI model that causes performance to degrade even when the model itself hasn't changed. In healthcare, this might occur when patient demographics, documentation practices, or disease patterns evolve away from the conditions the model was originally trained on.

**Data leakage**—The unintended exposure of sensitive information, such as when an AI model connected to your email inadvertently processes confidential data.

**Embeddings**—Mathematical representations (vectors) that encode the meaning of words or text in multidimensional space, allowing the model to turn relationships between concepts into computable mathematics.

**Frontier models**—The most advanced, highest-capability AI models available from leading vendors at any given time, typically reserved for paying subscribers.

**Generative AI**—Artificial intelligence that generates novel content—such as text, images, code, or audio—rather than simply retrieving or classifying existing information.

**Grounding**—The practice of anchoring an AI model's responses in specific source documents or retrieved data, rather than relying solely on patterns learned during training.

**Hallucination**—When an AI model confidently generates content that is factually incorrect or entirely fabricated, such as inventing a journal citation that does not exist.

**Health Insurance Portability and Accountability Act of 1996 (HIPAA)**—U.S. federal law that strictly limits how and when patient health data can be shared, imposing requirements on covered entities and their business associates.

**Large language model (LLM)**—A type of AI system trained on massive amounts of text that predicts the statistically most likely next word (token) in a sequence, enabling it to generate human-like text.

**Model collapse**—The degradation of AI model quality that occurs when new models are trained on AI-generated content rather than human-generated content.

**Model Context Protocol (MCP)**—A standardized protocol that provides a way for AI models to discover and use external tools and data sources, enabling richer integrations between AI systems and other software.

**Model drift**—Changes in an AI model's behavior over time as vendors update the underlying algorithms, potentially causing a prompt that worked reliably to start producing different or degraded outputs.

**Note bloat**—The inflation of clinical documentation length due to AI-generated text, templates, and autopopulated data, making it harder for subsequent readers to find the most clinically relevant information.

**Open-weight models**—AI models whose internal parameters (weights) are publicly available for anyone to download and run locally.

**Prompt engineering**—The skill of writing clear, structured instructions for generative AI systems to produce the desired output. Effective prompts often include a role, task, context, constraints, and format.

**Protected Health Information (PHI)**—Any individually identifiable health information held or transmitted by a covered entity or its business associate, protected under HIPAA.

**Retrieval-Augmented Generation (RAG)**—A technique that retrieves relevant documents from a defined corpus (such as clinical policies or the medical literature) and injects them into the model's context, grounding its answers in authoritative sources with a goal of reducing hallucinations.

**Safe Harbor**—A HIPAA de-identification method in which a specific list of identifiers is removed from a dataset, after which the data can be considered de-identified if no actual knowledge exists that remaining information could identify an individual.

**Shadow IT**—Hardware or software that employees use without the knowledge or approval of their organization's IT department, creating potential security and compliance risks.

**Summarization (compaction)**—The process by which an AI system condenses earlier portions of a long conversation into a shorter summary to make room for new messages within the context window.

**Synthetic feedback loop**—The risk that future AI models trained on AI-generated content (e.g., clinical documentation) will lose the nuance and intuition present in human-authored content.

**Temperature**—A model parameter that controls the randomness of output. Low temperature produces predictable, deterministic responses; high temperature produces more creative, varied responses.

**Tokens**—The units of language that LLMs process. A token can represent a whole word or a part of a word, and it may include punctuation. LLM usage is metered and charged by the token.

**Top-p (nucleus sampling)**—A model parameter that restricts the pool of candidate tokens to only those whose cumulative probability reaches a specified threshold, controlling the diversity of possible outputs.

**Transfer failure**—When an AI algorithm performs well in the environment where it was trained, but poorly when applied to a new environment with different patient demographics.

**Vectors**—Numerical coordinates in multidimensional space used to represent word meanings, enabling mathematical computation of language relationships.

**Vibe coding**—The practice of building software applications using natural-language prompts rather than manually writing traditional computer code.

**Zero Data Retention (ZDR)**—A policy in which the AI vendor processes your input solely to generate a response and does not log, store, or use it for model training afterward.

www.ingramcontent.com/pod-product-compliance
Lightning Source LLC
LaVergne TN
LVHW051059210926
848486LV00026B/430/J
* 9 7 9 8 9 9 5 8 4 0 2 0 6 *